Afraid of the Doctor

Afraid of the Doctor

Every Parent's Guide to Preventing and Managing Medical Trauma

Meghan L. Marsac

Melissa J. Hogan

ROWMAN & LITTLEFIELD
Lanham • Boulder • New York • London

This book represents reference material only. It is not intended as a medical manual, and the data presented here are meant to assist the reader in making informed choices regarding wellness. This book is not a replacement for treatment(s) that the reader's personal physician may have suggested. If the reader believes he or she is experiencing a medical issue, professional medical help is recommended. Mention of particular products, companies, or authorities in this book does not entail endorsement by the publisher or author.

Published by Rowman & Littlefield
An imprint of The Rowman & Littlefield Publishing Group, Inc.
4501 Forbes Boulevard, Suite 200, Lanham, Maryland 20706
www.rowman.com

6 Tinworth Street, London SE11 5AL, United Kingdom

British Library Cataloguing in Publication Information Available

Library of Congress Cataloging-in-Publication Data

Names: Marsac, Meghan L., 1981– author. | Hogan, Melissa J., 1973– author.
Title: Afraid of the doctor : every parent's guide to preventing and managing medical trauma / Meghan L. Marsac, Melissa J. Hogan.
Description: Lanham : Rowman & Littlefield, 2021. | Includes bibliographical references and index.
Identifiers: LCCN 2020058426 (print) | LCCN 2020058427 (ebook) | ISBN 9781538149188 (cloth) | ISBN 9781538149195 (epub)
Subjects: LCSH: Fear of doctors. | Children—Preparation for medical care. | Psychic trauma—Patients—Rehabilitation. | Sick children—Family relationships.
Classification: LCC R727.37 .M37 2021 (print) | LCC R727.37 (ebook) | DDC 616.85/2250083—dc23
LC record available at https://lccn.loc.gov/2020058426
LC ebook record available at https://lccn.loc.gov/2020058427

Contents

PART 3: WHO ARE YOU?

PART 4: STRATEGIES FOR PREVENTING AND REDUCING MEDICAL TRAUMA

PART 5: SPECIAL POPULATIONS

Foreword

> When health is absent, wisdom cannot reveal itself, art cannot become manifest, strength cannot be exerted, wealth is useless, and reason is powerless.
>
> —Herophilus, ancient Greek physician

I remember seeing her face when she came out of the first surgery. It was summer. Our then 16-year-old daughter Megan had just undergone a twelve-hour operation with a team of surgeons to address scoliosis due to her severe neuromuscular disorder known as Pompe disease. The curvature of her spine had gotten to be more than 100 degrees. During that first operation (there would be two more), the surgeons had begun to insert the screws into her vertebrae and had also attached a "halo" device to her head with screws drilled into her skull. Megan was unstable as they wheeled her out toward the intensive care suite. Her face was so swollen from lying face down during the surgery that she was unrecognizable. She looked like she had been, literally, hit by a truck.

Twelve hours earlier, my wife Aileen and I stood by Megan's side in the operating room, both fully sterilized and gowned up in scrubs. Megan looked stoically around the room. She acknowledged the remarkable team around her. We each held one of Megan's hands and fought with all of our might to hold back tears. We were not successful.

Just before the anesthesia flowed, Megan looked into our eyes and simply said, "It's okay. I got this." And with that, we felt a renewed strength. We needed it. We needed to be strong for each other. We needed to be strong for Megan's brothers. And we needed to be strong for her. We just didn't know how strong we would need to be in the two months ahead.

She would go on to have two more surgeries during that time. After the third surgery, finally back in her hospital room, her nurses quickly realized that the 25-year-old resident on duty, about a month out of medical school, had forgotten to order the post-surgery pain medication. It would take about 30 minutes for the medicine to come up from the pharmacy. Megan began to wail in agony. And I lost it. I was completely raw by the emotional drain and exhaustion of the prior seven weeks. I yelled loudly. At everyone. It was a complete meltdown.

And then in that moment, I felt a small hand touch mine. I looked down and it was Megan's. I was amazed that she had the strength to even move at all. She lightly grasped my hand and whispered, "It's okay, Daddy. I'll be fine. I just don't want you to be upset."

You could have heard a pin drop. And I thought to myself, "Who says these things? What strength does it take?"

Maybe that's the secret. Steel doesn't bend. It breaks. But it can be reinforced with other steel—in moments when you most need it, yet least expect it. For a parent, there is no greater pain than to see your child suffer. To see them filled with fear and anxiety. We all face it as parents of children going through medical challenges. And the kids themselves do as well. But in all of my 23+ years now in the world of unique medical challenges, watching children (including my own) suffer unimaginable procedures, traumas, pain and fear, what strikes me is how rare it is for them to feel sorry for themselves. They have a strength and perspectives that we big people are so often lacking.

I've long believed that the greatest trait that any person can have is empathy—to feel the hope, or the pain, of another. And to be there for them, for each other in a family and for your child. That's the secret—to acknowledge the reality and the costs of medical trauma on the whole family. And to be there to support one another despite those challenges. Maybe that's what is called, simply, love. And that is why this book is so important for any family going through a medical crisis or challenge. Where love meets medicine, indeed. . . .

John F. Crowley
Chairman and CEO, Amicus Therapeutics
Father of two children with Pompe disease
and one child with Asperger syndrome
February 28, 2021
World Rare Disease Day

Preface

Start where you are. Use what you have. Do what you can.

—Arthur Ashe

It always seems impossible until it is done.

—Nelson Mandela

Neither of us set out to write a book . . . but then life happened. We learned personally and professionally about the unique challenges of parenting children with medical conditions. We hope that by sharing our stories and writing this book, it will help your family as you navigate your own journey.

A NOTE FROM MELISSA

When I was a teenager, my mom tried to convince me to become a nurse. As a nurse herself, she told me about the rewards of helping people, the challenges of medicine, and the job opportunities.

I politely declined. Blood made me squeamish. So I became a lawyer instead.

I wanted 2.5 children, a house in the suburbs, and maybe a dog. I expected to have healthy children. Like many of us, I hoped my life would follow a certain path.

But life never goes exactly how we plan it.

Do I wish it had? Not really. And let me tell you why.

By the age of thirty-five, I'd had three children in a three-year period—all boys. I had my own business, and I felt like I was only a few lanes off of my original map for my life. But that would all soon change.

When my youngest son was two years old, he was diagnosed with a rare genetic condition called Hunter syndrome or mucopolysaccharidosis II. It's a long name for a terrible disease. The average life span is in the teens, after a child has slowly lost their mental and physical abilities. There is no cure.

I grieved intensely for about a year, although there was actually little time to grieve. My son started seeing medical specialists. He had several surgeries. He started a weekly infusion treatment that involved a full day at the hospital each week.

Every Wednesday night, I loaded up my car with toys, electronics, a stack of DVDs, and a wheelchair. I looked into the trunk and checked my list; I always seemed to forget something.

Preparing for a day at the hospital involved tangible planning, like packing the car and arranging childcare for my two other kids. It also involved emotional planning. I'd often shed a few tears, because despite all the preparation, it never felt normal to take my child to the hospital. My weary heart anticipated that, in all likelihood, the day would involve more than one needle poke, screaming, and a growing sense of loneliness I rarely shared with anyone.

Since my son was only two years old, he adapted for a while. *Until he didn't.*

I still remember the particular infusion visit where his veins collapsed three times. My son lost it. Kicking and screaming, it took an entire medical team to finish the infusion and get through the day.

That one disastrous visit turned into two. Two turned into three.

Appointments became all about how to manage his extreme feelings and reactions to everything the medical team was trying to do—things that *needed* to be done in order to treat his condition, things like IVs, anesthesia masks, needle pokes for infusions and blood draws, even blood pressure checks.

He refused to let people lift his shirt anymore for regular exams. He kicked and screamed as if he was being tortured. Using the anesthesia mask required five people to hold him down. Weekly needle sticks in his port-a-cath for infusions of his life-sustaining medication required someone to hold his arms and legs.

I was exhausted. And I was heartbroken because I wasn't sure what to do.

I didn't know what had happened to my son. He seemed so . . . *traumatized*.

At first, I didn't even know what to call what was happening. A friend mentioned the phrase *medical trauma*, and after some research, it felt so familiar. I scoured the Internet for more about what was going on with my son. I searched for and called experts. Could anyone help him?

Unfortunately for us, there was no one in our area who worked with cognitively impaired children, so I was on my own, with help from child life services at our local hospital. There was no child psychologist on staff.

I searched for a book to help me but couldn't find one. So I took notes. Managing my son's medical trauma became a part-time job, along with all the medical appointments he had. We accumulated lots of practice medical supplies (check out chapter 19 on desensitization and chapter 20 on medical play). We labeled all his procedures and appointments with short words or phrases he could understand (see chapter 15 on communication). He was given choices. Always.

For many years now, learning and putting into practice how to help my son manage his medical trauma has been a focal point of our journey. At some point, I also had to acknowledge and deal with my own emotions associated with the role I've played for many years in his medical care. I put on a happy face and work to make the medical world interesting and fun for him. But it's often an act.

On some days, I pat myself on the back. On other days, I cry in the car. But no matter what, I keep going. My son needs me.

The appointments still come and go. The surgeries, the infusions, the therapies, they're still with us. But now we face them from a place of knowledge and experience. We also look forward to the joyful moments, putting medical challenges in the context of our entire lives. After reading this book, I hope you can too.

LOOKING FOR ANSWERS

Although over time I learned to better manage my son's medical trauma challenges, I also continued to get questions from my son's disease community and other friends about medical trauma.

Medical trauma was a bigger problem than I had thought.

It turns out that millions of children develop medical trauma symptoms from their experience with medical procedures or appointments. And so do millions of parents.

As I continued to research, I kept seeing the name Dr. Meghan Marsac. I thought that maybe she could help untangle this trauma I saw developing in my son and in other children and families.

A NOTE FROM DR. MARSAC

A little bit about me: I always knew I wanted to work with kids. I loved their endless energy and interesting views of the world. I thought maybe I'd be a kindergarten teacher (but bulletin boards were not my friend) . . . maybe a pediatrician (but medical school did not sound fun) . . . maybe a kids' yoga instructor (but I trip over my own feet). As I explored all the ways in which I could have a fun job that helped bring out joy in children, I met Cody while volunteering at a hospital.

Cody was a three-year-old boy battling leukemia. His single mom was trying her best to juggle life and her child's treatment. As I visited with Cody at the hospital to give his mom some much-needed time to herself, his happiness and resilience captured my attention. I wondered how I could help him maintain such happiness and how I could better support his mother through this difficult time.

And so my journey to become a pediatric psychologist began. Now, years of school and life later, I have the privilege of partnering with families as they make their way through their medical journeys.

Early in my career, I had the opportunity to work with a bold and brave seven-year-old boy, Joey, who was battling a disease that resulted in recurrent tumors. Joey's medical team asked me to help with his difficult behaviors in clinic, including his refusal to have his port-a-cath accessed. The first time I watched his port access, both of his parents were yelling in frustration, Joey was thrashing around screaming and crying, and it took four nurses to hold him to give him his life-saving medication through his port. By the time his port access was finished, everyone in the room was exhausted and tense.

The family told me that this was getting worse every week. At every appointment, Joey was becoming angrier, and the family felt ready to give up. Joey's port access had become traumatic to him, even though, according to his medical team, "it wasn't supposed to hurt."

Together with Joey and his family, we came up with a new plan, adding one or two new strategies for the next three weeks. We applied the C.O.A.C.H. framework (more about this starting in chapter 2) by collecting information (why was port access difficult, what had worked in the past to help Joey overcome fears), observing (watching Joey's progress as we added new strategies), asking questions (asking the medical team how often port access was required, asking to have the same nurse work with Joey each week), choosing strategies (music as a distractor, creating a reward chart), and helping (getting help from multiple medical team members including the child life specialist, nurses, doctors, and psychologist).

After four weeks of working together, I watched Joey climb up on the exam table by himself and prepare himself for his port access. He put on his headphones to rock out to "Highway to Hell" (parent approved). Joey laid down calmly and got ready for his nurse (only one) to access his port. And he did it! He continued to bravely face his port access for the next year of treatment.

Since becoming a parent, I can more fully understand everything that we as health care providers ask parents to do to support their child's health. I have been blessed with two amazing, energetic boys, each of whom have had some run-ins with the medical world. I live the daily parenting juggle: the overwhelming love, joy, exhaustion, and general circus. And I must confess, I have looked at my own kids' doctors and thought, "You want me to do what? How can I possibly get my child to swallow that disgusting medicine? Have you tasted it?" My children have brought me opportunities to try out many of the strategies in this book, not only as a professional but also as a parent.

A lot of love and a little (okay, a lot of) patience are often the best tools to start with. You got this. You can do more than survive. You can thrive.

Acknowledgments

DR. MEGHAN MARSAC

This book is a passion project of mine—one that aims to help me reach my goal of making the medical world a better place for kids and their families.

I'd like to first thank my patients and their families, who inspire me and teach me daily: your strength and struggles drove me to write this book. Thank you for allowing me the privilege of being a part of your journeys and for sharing your worlds with me.

Thank you also to my mentors for encouraging me to walk my own path. I'd particularly like to thank Drs. Nancy Kassam-Adams, Melissa Alderfer, Lamia Barakat, Jeanne Brockmyer, Ethan Benore, and Flaura Winston, who have stuck with me over many years and taught me all about medical trauma and writing.

To the University of Kentucky, College of Medicine, and especially Drs. Scottie Day and Lindsay Ragsdale: thank you for your continued support and for encouraging me to write this book as a resource for the families we serve and beyond.

Thank you also to my coauthor, Melissa, who is one very talented, strong, persuasive, and determined woman. The decision to write this book with you was always a yes. To our agent, Steve Harris from CSG Literary Partners: thank you for recognizing the merit of this work. Thank you also to the dedicated team at Rowman & Littlefield, our publisher, for their work on this book.

I'd also like to thank Lori Sawicki, a fellow writer, who taught me the lay of the land and gave me all kinds of ideas and feedback on this book.

Thank you to my tribe, my amazing friends who show up with food, flowers, wrenches, texts, and phone calls when the going gets tough.

To my parents, Rita and Bob Guthrie, and brothers, Rich and Dave Guthrie, who always have my back, no matter what. And thank you, Mom, for reading this book even while recovering from surgery and taking care of everyone else . . . that's the thing about deadlines. And Dad, for fitting reading this book into an already crazy schedule.

And finally, to my children, James and Miles, who bring me more joy than I can describe and have redefined adventure in my life: You are totally awesome. Thank you for sharing our time together so I could write this book.

MELISSA J. HOGAN

I've always been a writer, starting with the book I wrote in eighth grade and continuing with the medical research articles I write now. I love writing, but it took me a long time and the support of a host of people to see that in myself, even though they saw it all along. I will be forever grateful to all of them.

To my children, Tyson, Brock, and Case, my grief is that your trauma was the impetus for this book. But sometimes out of ashes comes incredible beauty, and my hope for each of you is that what I've learned about trauma will continue to serve you and our relationships well in the years to come. I love you more than you will ever know.

Without the careful observation of Jane Hancock, my mother, who first suggested a diagnosis for my youngest son, I know this story would have turned out much differently. Thank you, Mom, for that and so much more. To my father, Ron Hancock, and to Oma Peg, thank you for all your support.

Although the last few years have been a storm, I could not have fared so well without the insight, support, and laughter of my brother Nate Hancock. You are a good man. And also to my brother Chris Hancock, my heart is with you.

Without the MPS community and the health care providers in it, I would not have started my journey investigating pediatric medical trauma. Jamie Fowler and Dr. Kendra Bjoraker specifically shared information and insight in those early challenging years. Special thanks goes to Dr. Joseph Muenzer and his team at the University of North Carolina Children's Hospital as well as the clinical research team at Vanderbilt Children's Hospital for their compassionate care for my son Case. Many thanks also to the team at Project Alive, who selflessly serve families on the path toward a cure for Hunter syndrome, and specifically the Dragon Moms, whose friendship is equal parts fire, wings, grief, and laughter.

To the therapists who have served me and my children: your knowledge and experience with trauma is a gift. We are safer and healthier because of you.

I am grateful to my colleagues in medical research, from those at the Food and Drug Administration to rare disease nonprofits to those in the pharmaceutical industry, who have grown more and more receptive to understanding how medical trauma can affect clinical trial participants and even the data as a result.

A very special thanks to all my writing friends and masterminds, especially to those who read and made suggestions to drafts of this book. Many thanks go to my coauthor, Dr. Meghan Marsac, for responding to an email from someone you didn't know about a topic in which you are a more respected expert than me. To our agent, Steve Harris from CSG Literary Partners, and the talented team at our publisher, Rowman & Littlefield: thank you for believing that this subject needed a voice on the shelves. To my SHOTS writers collective and fellow Hope*writers: thank you for your encouragement. Remember to write the books that your soul compels you to write. And to my writing mentors, Judge Alice Batchelder, Professor Teresa Brostoff, and Professor Alan Meisel: thank you for teaching me and believing in me.

Finally, there are those who have walked this challenging journey closely with me, those who sacrificed greatly and whose own stories may never be told. You know who you are. Your reward may not come in this lifetime, but hear it from me: thank you.

How to Use This Book

Very simply, the aim of this book is to support you in your efforts to help your child. We have written this book a bit like a reference guide, with stories and examples woven throughout. Names have been changed to protect patient privacy, but each story represents the experiences of actual families we've worked with or composites of such situations.

You can choose to read this book straight through, or you can jump to the sections that are most pressing for you and your family. If it is possible for you, we recommend reading it once from start to finish. Consider taking notes along the way or highlighting sections that you want to return to. Once you've gone through the book once, you can return to certain ideas or chapters as they come up in your child's journey.

Not everything in this book will be your experience today. Some things might come later on. Some symptoms or strategies might not apply to your family at all. Take what is helpful for you and leave the rest.

Part 1

THE REALITY OF MEDICAL TRAUMA

1

Where Love Meets Medicine

Some people care too much. I think it's called love.

—Winnie the Pooh

Jin sat quietly on the exam table in the doctor's office, her head down, feet slowly kicking back and forth. Her mom, Amy, watched her closely, remembering their last appointment—a visit that ended with Jin in tears, Amy with heartache watching her daughter's distress, and a nurse rushing out of the room.

Today, the door opened and the same nurse walked in. Amy noticed a flicker of recognition in her eyes. Amy knew from the nurse's tight, frozen smile that the nurse remembered Jin's last appointment as well.

Looking up, eyes wide, Jin didn't even try to smile. Instead, Amy watched her daughter's face fill with anxiety and fear.

Amy's heart was in a tug-of-war between the urge to protect her child from going through this again and the desire to hide in the corner until it was all over. But she knew the answer was really somewhere in the middle—she had to find a way to help Jin through this.

Amy's instincts are shared by many parents. As parents, we often have a natural urge to help our children through difficult circumstances. We balance this with the challenge of managing our own feelings and determining how much help to offer our children.

The powerful desire to protect our children can sometimes leave us feeling helpless. When dealing with medical procedures, this might be entirely new territory for us as parents. Medical challenges can feel like they are beyond the "typical" parenting challenges, but we can help our children face medical challenges, including medical trauma, using many of the parenting skills we already have.

CARING FOR OUR KIDS

The word *caring* literally means "feeling or showing concern for or kindness to others."[1]

We care about our children. We care about their health, their hopes, their future, their fears, and their feelings. We even care about them when they flop on the floor of the grocery store to express their true feelings through a tantrum or when they show us their best sass in their teenage years (really, we do care, even then!).

For many of us, from the moment we become parents, we care, but we also start to worry. Is my child eating enough? Growing enough? Learning enough? Are they getting picked on at school? Is my child choosing good friends? Are they getting into trouble? Of course, our concerns are likely reasonable at times. However, 61 percent of parents think that they can sometimes be overprotective.[2]

We can help our children face medical challenges, including medical trauma, using many of the same parenting skills we already have.

You can fill a bookshelf with parenting books that will address these typical parenting concerns and challenges. You can read a new book every week on a hot topic of today's most common parenting strategies. But facing medical challenges is unlike the more common parenting situations, and it can often feel unique and isolating. It may not be something your friends are talking about. The best-seller lists aren't full of books that help you navigate your child's medical challenges.

You care. Your child has a medical condition, an illness, or an injury. Our instinct is to fix it, to solve the problem. Medical treatment often takes time, unique expertise, and ongoing involvement with the health care system. As a parent, you want to help. But how?

WHERE'S MY INSTRUCTION MANUAL?

Children *should* come with an instruction manual. We don't drive a car without taking lessons, practicing, and taking a test, and parenting is infinitely more complex and important than driving. When we become a parent, we take a leap of faith. We often have little to no guidance when we start.

Parenting a child with a medical condition, genetic condition, or other health challenge often feels like it requires extra parenting skills. Sometimes it can feel like we need an advanced, superstar parenting class for these situations. But we can take what we already do and build on it.

A staggering number of families regularly have to manage health challenges involving their children. In other words, though your journey may feel lonely at times, millions of other parents walk similar paths. Approximately 40 percent of children in the United States suffer from a chronic health problem.[3] For example,

- six million U.S. children have asthma,[4]
- fifteen million U.S. children are living with rare diseases,[5]
- fifteen thousand U.S. children are newly diagnosed with cancer each year,[6] and
- tens of millions of children require treatment for injuries every year.[7]

Children with chronic health conditions are at increased risk for emotional and behavioral problems.[8,9] Parents of children with chronic health conditions also often experience physical and psychological health challenges.[10,11] So how do we prepare ourselves for that risk—or in many cases, that reality?

How can we maintain or improve our child's health and development without feeling like we are going crazy in the process?

In addition to using regular parenting skills to help our children deal with medical challenges and tough feelings, we might need to gather some additional information or add new skills to our parenting toolbox. Parents of children with medical needs often benefit from learning about their child's condition as well as related topics.

It is helpful for parents of children with medical conditions or significant medical challenges to learn

- about their child's medical condition or challenge,
- what information to share with their child,
- how to share information with their child,
- how to help their child deal with this information,
- how to maximize their organization skills to manage medical treatment along with life,
- how to make medical decisions (sometimes with an overwhelming amount of information and sometimes with very little information),
- how to help their child deal with medical procedures and medications,
- how to adapt to ever-changing situations,
- how to help their child deal with ever-changing situations, and
- how to become an advocate for their child.

This book is designed to guide you through developing specialized parenting skills to support your child through health challenges. Managing medical trauma (i.e., the emotional reactions to medical conditions/treatment) is often a part of those challenges.

HELP ON THE JOURNEY

When we add knowledge and skills to our desire to help our child, we strengthen our ability to help them.

For each child and each family situation, helping may look different. There are some supports that most everyone needs: general emotional support, respite care (someone to look after the child so parents can have a break), and advocacy for their child and family. For many families, the added complication of medical trauma requires even more support.

In this book, *medical trauma* refers to the emotional impact of children's health conditions and/or medical treatment. Medical trauma can affect *any* family member—the child with a health condition, a typically developing sibling (a sibling without a health condition), a parent, a grandparent, or other family members.

As defined by the National Child Traumatic Stress Network, medical trauma is "a set of psychological and physiological responses of children and their families to pain, injury, serious illness, medical procedures, and invasive or frightening treatment experiences."[12] In other words, the challenges of living with and managing health conditions extend to emotional health as well.

Throughout this book, we present the journeys of four families who have a child with health challenges. You will meet Cameron, Nia, Daniel, and Jin. You might see a little bit of your own child in one or more of their stories, or your child's situation may feel completely unique.

Meet Cameron

Cameron, a thirteen-year-old boy, joins us one week after being involved in a car accident. His father was driving. Cameron sustained multiple injuries in the accident, including two broken legs that required emergency surgery. He spent the first week after the accident in the hospital and is expecting to go home in another week. He will likely have additional surgeries and a lengthy rehabilitation. Cameron lives with his parents, Zoe and Preston, and younger brother, Emerson. Cameron tries to avoid talking about the car crash and has frequent nightmares.

Meet Nia

We meet Nia, an eight-year-old girl battling rhabdomyosarcoma (a type of cancer), six months into her treatment. Nia struggles to cooperate with her medical team. She has a severe fear of needles. She lives with her mother, Maria, and older sister, Sara.

Meet Daniel

Daniel is a three-year-old boy diagnosed with Hunter syndrome—a rare genetic condition that affects physical, social, and emotional development. Hunter syndrome can involve behaviors similar to autism spectrum disorder, attention deficit hyperactivity disorder, and sensory processing disorder. We meet Daniel four months after his diagnosis. Daniel lives with his grandparents, whom he calls Nana and Papa. His mother, Sandy, placed him in his grandparents' care shortly after learning of his diagnosis. Daniel's mother was afraid she wouldn't be able to manage the intensity of the treatments that he would need. She knew his grandparents would be able to support him.

Meet Jin

Jin is a four-year-old girl, adopted from China, whom we meet as she struggles through vaccinations in her pediatrician's office. We later follow Jin on a trip to the emergency room related to high blood sugar. She lives with her adoptive mother, Amy, and father, Cole.

The goal of sharing these stories and this book is to offer a guide to help you as you navigate your family's own journey. We also hope to help you identify your existing strengths as a parent and the unique challenges in your child's health journey. Finally, we hope you will use this book to build skills to add to your natural parenting strengths. With these new skills, you will be better equipped to shape your child's and your own journey over time.

QUESTIONS TO ASK YOURSELF

- How would I describe my parenting journey so far?
- What part of parenting brings me joy?
- What are my biggest parenting success stories?
- What tips would I have for someone who is parenting a child with a similar medical journey?
- What do I want to get from reading this book?

ACTION STEPS

- Set up a notebook to use for notes about your child and family as you read this book. Use this notebook when you respond to the Action Steps sections. A binder that you can add to or remove pages from works well for this. We will refer to this notebook as your C.O.A.C.H. notebook. We'll talk more about the C.O.A.C.H. process starting in the next chapter.
- In your notebook, write down your three biggest parenting challenges right now.

- Identify the people who help you emotionally, physically, and financially (your support system), and jot them down in your C.O.A.C.H. notebook.
- Identify the people who help your child or children emotionally, physically, and financially (their support system), and include them in your notebook.

2

Parenting through Medical Challenges

Why her?

—Parent of an eleven-year-old with cancer

It is easier to build strong children than to repair broken men.

—Frederick Douglass

Before you had a child, did you ever say to yourself, "When I have kids, *I'll* do _____"? Or "I won't do things *that* way"? Sometimes it feels like there is a magical parenting formula. But then a few years into parenting, we usually realize things don't always go as planned.

Take a minute to think about your current goals as a parent. Have they changed since your child experienced health challenges or was diagnosed with a medical or genetic condition?

Parents are key to their child's medical journey.

Parents are key to their child's medical journey. Parents serve as managers, caregivers, entertainers, coaches, rule makers, and cheerleaders. You name it, and you are probably doing it. As a parent, you can help shape your child's experience throughout their life and medical journey.

You are often the main lens through which your child sees their situation. Is it scary? Is it weird? Is it an adventure? How you decide to approach parenting can directly affect how your child responds to medical situations. But, as every parent knows, kids have minds of their own. Even when you have done a dynamite job at supporting your child, sometimes things still do not go smoothly.

While parenting is a great responsibility and a huge challenge, it is also a great opportunity.

WHAT'S MY PARENTING STYLE?

Knowing how you tend to parent overall can help you choose the most natural strategies to help your child with their medical condition and treatment.

Parenting styles can be characterized as authoritative, authoritarian, permissive, or uninvolved.[1,2] While not all parents fit squarely within one category, your instincts often lead you toward one over the others in how you parent.

If you parent with an authoritative style, you try to influence your child by explaining the reasons behind the rules while also listening to your child's reasoning. You hold some rules strongly in place but may also change certain rules. You generally encourage your child's independence, but you balance that with their need to follow the rules.

If you parent with an authoritarian style, you likely have very strict rules and use punishment to encourage your child to behave as you expect them to. You generally limit your child's independence and focus instead on instilling respect and obedience.

If you're the opposite of authoritarian, you might parent with a permissive style. In this parenting style, you tend to follow your child's lead and make few demands of them. Permissive parents often allow their child to direct themselves and their family. If you're a permissive parent, you might notice that you avoid imposing much structure on your child.

Finally, there is the uninvolved parent. This type of parent doesn't try to actively engage with their child and may not be present emotionally and/or physically. This is unlikely to be you, since you're investing in your child and their situation by reading this book, but you might have a spouse or coparent who is uninvolved.

Knowing your tendencies as a parent will help you select strategies that fit your family and each individual child. For example, let's say that you are having a problem getting your child to take their medication. Every time you get the pill, syringe, or shot ready, you may feel your own anxiety increasing as you know your child will fight it. If you prefer to give your child more freedom and guide the way, you may not want to jump to implementing a structured behavioral management plan (we will explain what this is in chapter 17). Instead, you may want to try medical play first (see chapter 20). You may want to give your child choices about when or how to take their medication. However, if medical play isn't working, you may want to try another strategy, such as creating a more structured plan for your child.

Knowing your child helps you choose effective parenting strategies. If you have more than one child, you may have already experienced the difference in how children respond to the same kind of rules or discipline. For example, let's say that you provided a consequence of time-out when your child hit their nurse. One child might break down in tears, sobbing that they didn't mean to and they're so sorry. Another child will look you right in the eyes and say, "I don't care!" As you explore the strategies in this book, consider yourself, your child, and each situation when deciding what will work best for your family.

HOW TO BE YOUR CHILD'S C.O.A.C.H.

As we mentioned at the beginning of this chapter, you are key to your child's medical journey. If they are the main character, you are the director, producer, and set designer. If they are the lead singer, you are the sound engineer, guitarist, and drummer. If they are the star pitcher, you are their *coach*.

When we thought about the coach concept, we realized that it really reflected what parents are trying to do to help their child succeed. This is especially true for situations that are uniquely challenging, such as medical trauma.

We developed a guide that you can use as you consider your child's unique situation and how best to help them—how to C.O.A.C.H. them:

Collect information.
Observe the situation.
Ask questions of yourself, your child, and professionals.
Choose your strategies.
Help your child, and get help from others.

In a nutshell, this book will walk you through how to C.O.A.C.H. your child through medical challenges and medical trauma.

As you C.O.A.C.H. your child, you are also modeling and teaching them to do the same for themselves. This is especially important if they have a lifelong condition.

Let's jump in and take a step toward applying our C.O.A.C.H. process to our friends Nia and Daniel.

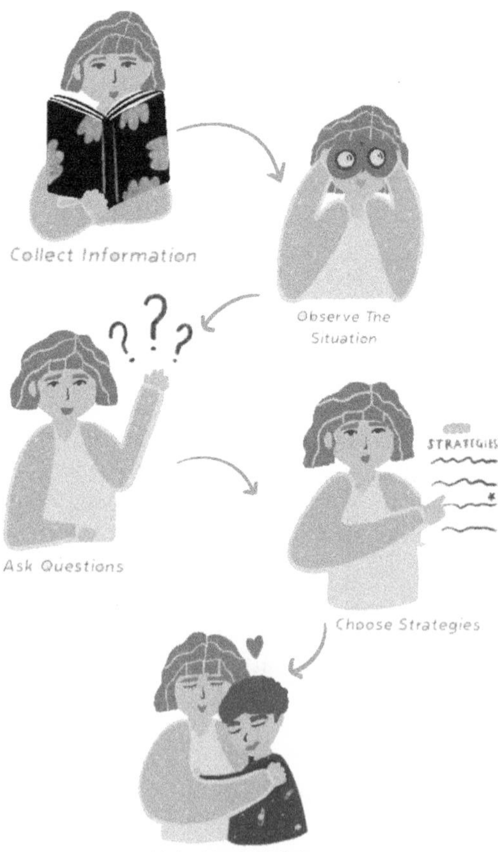

Figure 2.1.
The C.O.A.C.H. Process

Helping Nia Take Her Medications

Nia's mother, Maria, tends toward a child-centered, more permissive parenting style. She values her children's opinions. She allows Nia to make many decisions. For example, she lets Nia choose to go to bed when she is tired rather than establishing a standard bedtime. Recently, however, Maria's natural parenting style has been conflicting with some of Nia's required medical treatment.

According to Nia's doctors, she needs to take medications on a very specific schedule. It's been difficult for Maria to get Nia to take her medications on time. Maria spends lots of time each day negotiating and convincing Nia to take her medications.

During clinic visits, the medical team also expects Nia to cooperate quickly. This places more pressure on both Maria and Nia.

Frustrated with all the time she is spending negotiating with Nia, Maria asks Nia why she immediately becomes upset when it's time to take her medicine. She asks Nia what scares her about her appointments. Nia struggles a bit to identify her fears and can't really explain why she hates her medications—she just does. Maria continues to listen to Nia. She observes her when she struggles. Over time, Maria and Nia figure out that not knowing what to expect, being surprised, and being rushed are difficult for Nia. Also, Nia tries to forget about the cancer. Taking her medications reminds her that she is sick, and the rigid schedule makes her feel pressured to do things *right away*.

While Maria chooses to maintain her permissive style in many aspects of parenting, she seeks out guidance to create a more directive, structured approach to getting Nia to take her medications. It takes Nia a few days to accept these new strategies, but Maria sticks with it. They are able to greatly improve Nia's experience taking medication.

If you look at the C.O.A.C.H. process, Maria *collected* information from her daughter and her medical team. She made sure she understood their expectations about the medications. She learned more about what the visits would require of Nia.

Maria *observed* that Nia struggled in shifting from self-directing much of her activity to being told what to do regarding medications and appointments.

Maria *asked* herself what she could do differently, she asked Nia why she was struggling and how she could help, and she asked the medical team what they could change and how much leeway they had with medications and appointments.

Maria *chose* to start with a visual and reward-based strategy that required more structure in taking medications. She also chose to help Nia understand and better prepare for appointments ahead of time.

Maria was able to *help* Nia by working her plan and being consistent with it. This helped Nia feel safe and supported.

Helping Daniel with New Medical Fears

Daniel's grandparents tend toward an authoritative approach. They try to explain to Daniel why he needs certain medications. They try to help him communicate his feelings and work with him to plan for his procedures. Nana and Papa had been helping care for Daniel since he was a baby, and he had previously done very well with his medical appointments and procedures. However, a few months after starting weekly infusions, he needed to be carried into the clinic because he was so upset.

Several weeks later, his grandparents noticed that even before they reached the hospital, Daniel started getting anxious. As they got out of the car, Daniel pulled on Papa's arm and started repeating, "No, no, no."

After learning more about different strategies for supporting Daniel, his grandparents decide to try a couple of different approaches. They work with Daniel to create a routine with a picture schedule to follow at each appointment (see chapter 18). They create a reward system to use during each infusion (see chapter 17). They also use a more child-centered approach by providing Daniel with the opportunity to use medical play at home (see chapter 20).

If we review the C.O.A.C.H. process, Daniel's grandparents *collected* information for many years—years in which his medical appointments had gone well. They knew what to expect.

They *observed* a change in Daniel's behaviors. Daniel showed new reactions to coming to the hospital and to what he was experiencing there. They started to see things how he might see them—the white coats, the nurses rushing about, the crying in the next room.

Nana and Papa *asked* the hospital what reward systems they had for children who were often at the hospital. They asked friends what systems they used for their children. They also asked the hospital for some extra medical supplies that they could use in medical play to simulate an infusion with Daniel's stuffed animals at home.

They *chose* to implement a reward system, visual schedule, and some medical play strategies, and they maintained consistency.

These strategies *helped* Daniel slowly overcome his fears about his infusions.

QUESTIONS TO ASK YOURSELF

- What parenting or personal strengths do I bring to my child's current medical care and health challenges?
- In what recent situation could I award myself superstar parent status?
- What hasn't gone well lately? What might I need to change to help my child differently in the future?
- What is unique about my child that might influence how I support them?

ACTION STEPS

- Thinking about your child's most recent medical appointment, write down in your notebook how you used or could have used the C.O.A.C.H. process.
- Identify the person or people in your support system who help you C.O.A.C.H. your child and make note of it in your notebook.
- Write down any of your thoughts from the questions section above that you want to remember or follow up on.

3

The Medical Journey

Alice: Would you tell me, please, which way I ought to go from here?

The Cheshire Cat: That depends a good deal on where you want to get to.

—Lewis Carroll, *Alice in Wonderland*

I'm not telling you it's going to be easy—I'm telling you it's going to be worth it.

—Art Williams

No doubt you've heard the phrase "two steps forward, one step back." Medical journeys are a bit like that. Except maybe add a "slide to the left" here, a "do-si-do" there, moving forward, then backward, maybe in a circle, often with a blurry destination or an ever-changing target.

We'd like to believe there's a sign pointing straight back to "normal" and that it's just around the next bend. That's not to say that medical challenges will always be part of your life or that they'll always be hard. But more often than not, the path to get there is a winding one.

It might look something like figure 3.1.

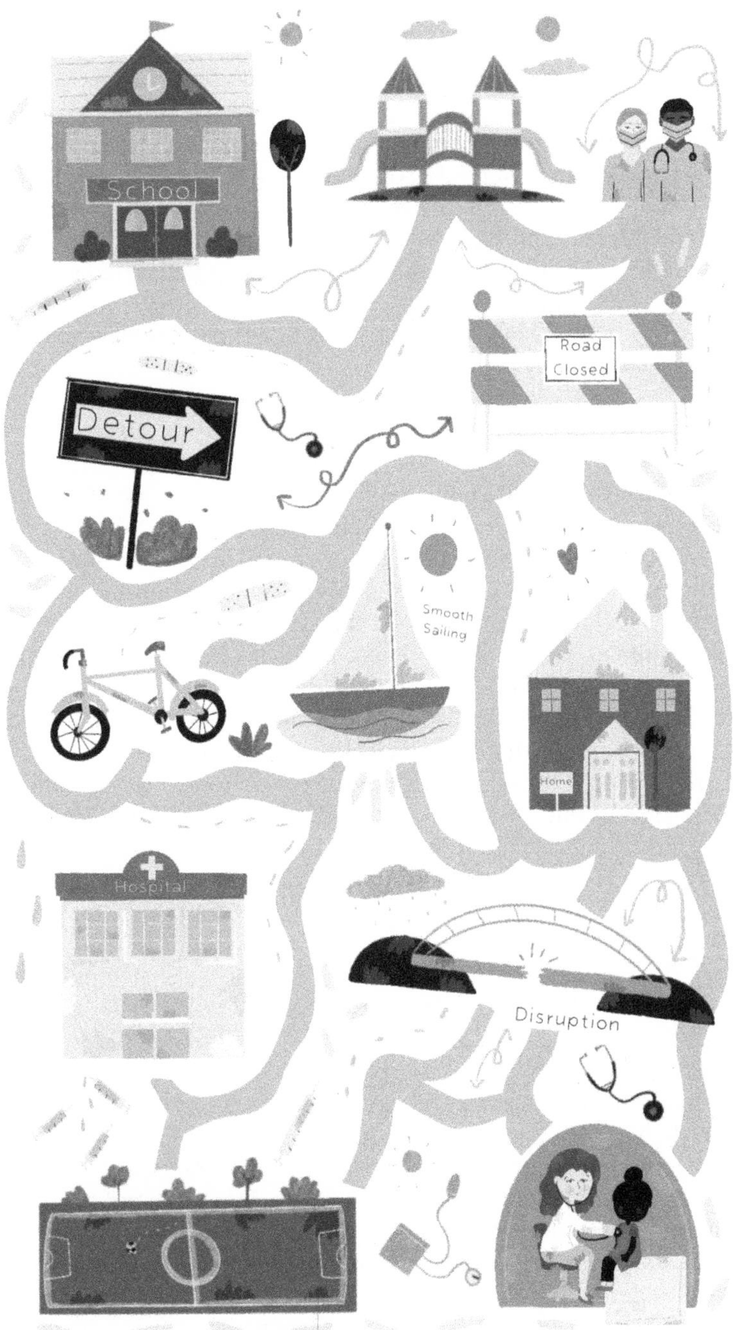

Figure 3.1. A Medical Journey

As a first step in supporting your child (and yourself), take a minute to stop and think about where your child, you, and your family are on your child's medical journey. Consider where you've been in the past and where you might still feel lost. Ask yourself where you want to go.

Taking the time to recognize your family's strengths and challenges can be helpful as you plan how to manage your child's ongoing medical journey.

Let's look at some of our families and how they might view their own medical journeys.

Cameron's Early Journey

We meet Cameron early in his medical journey, one week after a car accident resulted in serious injuries. In the first weeks following his injuries, it's not surprising that Cameron and his family members are having intense emotional reactions. Cameron's mother, Zoe, is Cameron's main support person; she is helping him through his early treatment and does not leave his side. Zoe recognizes that Cameron is having difficulty with medical care, and she is trying everything to support him. She asks his doctors about his emotional reactions and is told that they are normal following a serious injury.

At this point in the journey, Cameron's father, Preston, is battling his own guilt about the accident; even though he was not at fault for the car crash, he can't help but feel responsible. Preston is unable to visit Cameron frequently in the hospital—he needs to go back to work, but that also makes a good excuse to avoid the hospital and his pangs of guilt.

Back at home, Cameron's brother, Emerson, is staying with grandparents, who are trying to keep his schedule normal. While Emerson is missing his parents and is worried about his brother, he feels strongly supported by his grandparents. Zoe calls Emerson every night to check in, and his grandparents bring him to visit on the weekend.

There are many people involved in Cameron's medical journey, so we can already see that it won't be a straight path from A to B. Cameron is also still near the beginning of his journey. The intense emotions of the accident still make it hard for the family members to come together on a plan or a path. While Zoe is already implementing some of the C.O.A.C.H. strategies (collecting information, observing, and asking questions), the strategies to help Cameron at this stage may be different than those needed a month from now, much less three months from now.

C.O.A.C.H. is not a linear process. Sometimes you collect information, ask questions, then go back and collect more information. Sometimes you choose a strategy, observe new behaviors, go back and ask more questions, and then choose another strategy.

Jin's Journey

When we first meet Jin, she is struggling with needle sticks for her vaccinations at her pediatrician's office. As Jin was adopted, we are unsure where her medical journey began. Her adoptive parents' journey specific to Jin's health begins with the challenges in her pediatrician's office. The path continues to unfold during a trip to the emergency room after a blood sugar check in the pediatrician's office reveals an extremely high blood sugar level. At the emergency room, Jin is inconsolable. She fights exams by members of the medical team, and they struggle to insert an IV.

Jin is ultimately diagnosed with type 1 diabetes. The doctor who diagnoses Jin also mentions to Amy that Jin is not talking at the level she would expect of a four-year-old. The doctor asks Amy and Cole a few more questions about Jin's development, trying to understand if what she is seeing might be a current symptom of her diabetes or a separate issue. The doctor ultimately recommends that Jin's parents take her for a speech and occupational therapy evaluation. The doctor explains to Jin's parents that she might be having trouble in the ER and at her other medical appointments because she might not be able to understand what is happening. Also, changes in blood sugar can affect mood, which could make Jin more tired or more irritable at times. Given that Jin's diabetes will require many more medical appointments, the family knows they need to figure out how to help her with her reactions in medical environments.

This moment is a huge turning point for Jin's family. Their journey has detoured in a new and unexpected direction. They now have an additional unknown about Jin's ability to communicate. However, now Amy and Cole can make a plan to help Jin with her diabetes and figure out how to support her communication.

As we'll learn in part 4 of this book, on specific strategies for preventing and managing medical trauma, communication is key.

Communication challenges have the potential to contribute to medical trauma. It can be very stressful when a child is unable to understand or process what is happening *around* them and *to* them. That makes it difficult to walk the medical journey *with* them.

QUESTIONS TO ASK YOURSELF

- How did my family's medical journey begin?
- What have been the biggest challenges along the way?
- How have my child and I overcome challenges that we've each faced?
- What setbacks are each of us currently facing? How can we address them?

ACTION STEPS

- In your C.O.A.C.H. notebook, draw a map of your child's medical journey until now.
- Add possible paths that your child's medical journey could take in the future.
- Make a list of everything that currently feels overwhelming about your child's medical journey.

Part 2

MEDICAL TRAUMA 101

4

What Exactly Is Medical Trauma?

> My daughter is so petrified; she's terrified of needles. I don't know where that came from. She wasn't afraid of needles. . . . Now, she's terrified of needles.
>
> —Parent of an eleven-year-old girl with cancer

> Trauma creates change you don't choose. Healing is about creating change that you do choose.
>
> —Michele Rosenthal, post-traumatic stress disorder survivor

Medical trauma, post-traumatic stress disorder, medical post-traumatic stress disorder, post-traumatic stress symptoms, post-trauma psychological sequalae, medical traumatic stress, pediatric medical traumatic stress, and medical anxiety: these are all terms used to describe the emotional and physiological (that is, changes in the body) reactions that many children with medical conditions and their family members experience. These reactions can happen when a child is diagnosed with a medical condition, undergoes medical treatment, and/or has a change in prognosis of their medical condition. In this book, we use the term *medical trauma* to describe these types of reactions.

As we noted earlier in the book, the National Child Traumatic Stress Network defines medical trauma as "a set of psychological and physiological responses of children and their families to pain, injury, serious illness, medical procedures, and invasive or frightening treatment experiences."[1] In other words, children who have medical conditions face many challenges related to the condition itself, treatment, and treatment side effects. These challenges can affect how they feel and how their body responds. Other family members may also experience similar changes in the way they feel and in how their body responds to these experiences.

Medical trauma reactions can be similar to reactions that children and adults experience when they are exposed to other types of trauma. Most commonly, when people hear about "trauma" or "post-traumatic stress disorder," the first image that comes to mind is that of a veteran who has been exposed to trauma during their military service. Military veterans' experiences and trauma reactions were among the first types of trauma to be recognized by the medical field.

A common example of a post-traumatic stress disorder reaction involves a veteran hearing a car backfire and dropping to the ground thinking it is a gunshot. In war, this is an instinctive response that can actually save their life; in war, dropping to the ground when you hear gunfire is helpful and adaptive. However, if you are in a safe place, dropping to the ground when you hear a similar sound is an overreaction and is unhelpful. This may actually cause more distress. The body can become misprogrammed based on a traumatic experience. Children with medical conditions and their family members can experience similar misprogramming.

Children who have medical conditions face many challenges related to the condition itself, treatment, and treatment side effects.

Post-traumatic stress disorder develops based on exposure to situations that we perceive as very scary and possibly life-threatening.[2] Our mind and body continue to perceive a threat even when the physical threat is gone. Sometimes this perception is in our mind and awareness; other times the memories are in our body and not in our conscious awareness. When faced with a threat, whether it is a real threat in the moment or a perceived threat based on our past experience, our body prepares to physically fight the threat or run away from the threat. In some cases, we also freeze in the face of the threat. This is commonly referred to as the "fight-flight-freeze" response.[3]

Children with medical conditions can experience fight, flight, freeze, or a combination of these if they are afraid during medical care. A fight response could include crying, clenching fists or jaw, yelling, arguing with doctors, or becoming physically aggressive with medical providers (e.g., kicking, hitting, biting). Examples of flight responses include refusing to look at providers, trying to run out of the treatment room, or trying to wiggle away when they need to be still for a medical procedure. Finally, examples of a freeze response could include a child holding their breath, zoning out, or watching everyone closely without communicating. A child who is freezing up may not be able to answer questions or tell their parents or medical providers what they need (e.g., if they are feeling pain or if they don't understand what is happening).

Children with medical conditions can experience fight, flight, freeze, or a combination of these if they are afraid during medical care.

When a true threat is present, the fight-flight-freeze response can be beneficial. In the earlier example, in a warzone, dropping to the ground when there is a loud noise has a purpose—to protect yourself from the threat. However, sometimes our bodies get stuck in this reaction. We react as if there is a threat present based on our emotional trauma. Medical trauma reactions are based on this same feeling of threat—regardless of whether or not an actual threat is present. Similar to a war veteran unconsciously fearing the sound of a gunshot, a child with medical trauma may unconsciously fear a room or a certain procedure that previously went poorly (see chapter 5 to learn about specific medical trauma symptoms).

Sometimes even children without chronic medical conditions can develop medical trauma reactions related to routine medical care. Does your child worry for days about shots at the doctor's office? Are they afraid to go to the dentist, even for a cleaning?

Both children and parents alike might wonder if they are the only ones feeling this way, asking themselves questions like, "What is wrong with me? Am I crazy? Does this happen to anyone else?" These feelings and questions are common. The quick answers are, "Nothing is wrong with you. No, you are not crazy. And yes, this happens to many children and parents." While many children and parents experience these challenges, there are options that can help you feel better. We'll talk about them in this book. And even more help is out there if you need it.

How many people experience these types of reactions? The short answer is millions. Nearly one out of every three children with medical conditions, their siblings, and their parents experience significant medical trauma.[4] "Simple" vaccinations are the most common medical procedure experienced by children worldwide,[5] and they commonly cause children significant anxiety and distress.[6] Over 60 percent of children report fears about needles.[7] Approximately 40 percent of children report significant fears about going to the dentist.[8]

What causes medical trauma? We don't know all the answers yet. But what we do know is that when a child or family member feels scared about a new diagnosis, prognosis, or treatment, they are more likely to have medical trauma reactions.[9]

Anyone who is going through medical treatment can develop medical trauma, even when appointments are considered routine.

Surprisingly, it doesn't matter if someone has a medical condition that is "severe." Anyone who is going through medical treatment can develop medical trauma, even when appointments are considered routine (such as vaccinations at your child's pediatrician's office). However, the more of these tough, frightening experiences someone has, the more likely they are to experience medical trauma. But it can also happen after experiencing only one scary event.

When does medical trauma happen? Sometimes it is obvious and appears right after a scary new diagnosis or a bad experience with medical treatment. Other times medical trauma can sneak up on us, building slowly and then suddenly feeling overwhelming.

Research suggests that it is a combination of many factors that make it more likely for someone to experience medical trauma.[10,11] Medical trauma is more common if someone

- experiences their medical condition or treatment as life-threatening,
- has been exposed to other traumatic events,
- has less support from their family and/or community,
- uses certain types of coping, such as avoidance (read more about that in the next chapter),
- is female (studies suggest that females are at a higher risk for medical trauma), or
- already has emotional health challenges before a medical event.

While these factors make it more likely, medical trauma can still happen to anyone.

In chapter 5, we will talk more about the specific signs and symptoms of medical trauma.

Medical Trauma in Jin

Jin continues to fight during her wellness checks at her pediatrician's office. She also fought the doctors and her parents in the emergency room as she was being diagnosed with diabetes.

As Jin interacts more and more with the health care system, she starts to develop medical trauma reactions. Although her pediatrician recognizes that Jin is having communication difficulties (which can make things scarier), her provider is not fully aware of how each new medical appointment is affecting Jin. Because it is hard for Jin to communicate her feelings, it is also difficult for her family and medical providers to recognize that she is not fighting because she is being oppositional or difficult; she is fighting because she is afraid.

Jin's care is not limited to traditional medical providers. She is now also seeing a speech therapist for her communication challenges. At first, adding a speech therapy appointment to Jin's schedule triggers similar fighting responses in Jin. This reminds Jin of her other medical appointments and interactions, which sometimes include painful procedures like shots or needle sticks to check her blood sugar. But luckily for Jin's family, the speech therapist recognizes Jin's responses as medical trauma and suggests that Jin and her family see a mental health provider to help them learn how to manage her challenging behaviors.

Once Jin's parents have a better understanding that her behaviors are related to her fears and difficulty communicating those fears, they are able to take a whole new approach to supporting Jin through her medical appointments.

QUESTIONS TO ASK YOURSELF

- How do I react to a medical procedure or when I receive new health information about my child? Why do I react that way?
- Has my child ever shown confusing behaviors during a medical appointment?

ACTION STEPS

- In your C.O.A.C.H. notebook, make a list of behaviors or reactions that your child exhibits when they are worried or nervous about something. Circle the reactions that your child has during medical care or when they are worried about their health.
- Make a list of your own reactions when you are worried about something. Circle reactions that you have had related to your child's medical condition or care.

5

How Do I Know if My Child Has Medical Trauma?

> I think [the hardest part of treatment] for him is the anticipation of what's coming next. . . . If he knows something's going to happen Friday, he'll start worrying about it two days before.
>
> —Parent of an eight-year-old child with cancer

Many of the examples in this book might make medical trauma seem obvious. As we initially described in Jin's story, she was crying and fighting at her medical appointments. Though her parents may not have known that her reactions are part of something called "medical trauma," they were able to recognize that she had developed fears of hospitals and doctors.

Sometimes medical trauma reactions are much harder to identify, and many people are not aware of medical trauma at all. These reactions can be underrecognized in kids with medical conditions.[1] Medical trauma can show up in different ways in different children and families. Maybe something about your child just seems off. You can't quite put your finger on it. Maybe your child has changed from being super energetic to a little more down. Or maybe they could usually control their feelings, but now it seems like little things can set them off.

Medical trauma can show up in different ways in different children and families.

Similarly, a coparent might snap at you when you ask questions about your child's medical care, or your spouse might be "too busy" to attend medical appointments. Your child, your child's siblings, and other family members can each have medical trauma. It can look different in every person.

In this chapter, we will focus on medical trauma in children, but see chapters 30, 31, and 32 for information about medical trauma in caregivers.

Symptoms of medical trauma can be grouped into several categories, including changes in overall mood, symptoms of reexperiencing, symptoms of hyperarousal, and symptoms of avoidance.[2]

CHANGES IN OVERALL MOOD

Changes in mood are just that: a change in your child's typical mood. Some children become more withdrawn. This can look like keeping to themselves more, withdrawing from friends or family, or starting to interact less with their doctors or nurses. Other children might become more worried or anxious about medical appointments or their health or about life in general. Some kids become more sad, angry, irritable, or snappy.

Sometimes the mood change is clear: you are getting ready to go to the doctor's office and your child is suddenly sensitive or angry. Other times your child's mood change might seem entirely unrelated to their medical condition. For example, they may suddenly become very impatient with their brother for taking their favorite toy, or they may start yelling at you for not having their favorite shirt clean. Or your child may start spending a lot more time alone in their room.

Symptoms of medical trauma can be grouped into several categories, including changes in overall mood, reexperiencing, hyperarousal, and avoidance.

These behaviors could be signs of many different challenges, such as typical sibling disagreements, a developmental stage, hormones, or reactions to everyday circumstances. While one or more of those might be the case, these reactions also could be a sign of medical trauma.

REEXPERIENCING

Symptoms of reexperiencing can manifest in various ways. In children, we often see it come out in their play: they may draw pictures of a medical procedure or play with toys reenacting a doctor's appointment. They may become distressed when engaging in medical play.

Reexperiencing can also take the form of bad dreams. Some children have scary dreams directly related to their medical condition or treatment; others have more general bad dreams.

Children might repetitively talk or write about their medical condition or a particularly scary procedure and have a hard time getting it out of their mind. Some children might feel like thoughts about their injury event or medical condition are stuck in their head; they keep trying to think about other things, but they can't. All these reactions can be normal and beneficial; however, they can also be signs of medical trauma.

Many children show increased worries or anxiety at night and may need more comfort or support from parents. Children might have trouble getting scary thoughts out of their mind so that they can fall asleep.

Each of these symptoms can be a sign of medical trauma.

HYPERAROUSAL

Hyperarousal is generally experienced in the body. This is the trauma symptom that is most related to the fight-flight-freeze response that we discussed in chapter 4.

A bit more on the fight-flight-freeze response: this is where your body prepares to stay and fight off a threat, run away to escape the threat, or becomes paralyzed by the threat. Imagine how you would feel if you were out on a hike and a grizzly bear was headed your way. Do you pick up a stick to fight it off? Do you run the other way? Or maybe you shake in your boots and cannot, for the life of you, move an inch.

Faced with a grizzly bear, your heart would likely start racing to pump blood to your muscles. You would start to breathe faster. You might start to sweat. You might get dizzy. Your sympathetic nervous system would be activated. When our body responds in this way to an actual immediate threat, it gives us the energy and strength that we need for survival. When the body has a *hyperarousal* response (i.e., is activated when it doesn't need to be), it gets stuck in the fight-flight-freeze place—even when the threat is gone.

At times, children experience their medical treatment or medical condition as a threat. They can then get stuck in their fight-flight-freeze response. Sometimes this response can be retriggered when a child is reminded of a fear. Sometimes we see this in our children's vital signs. Has your child's blood pressure or pulse ever been elevated at a medical appointment when there seemed to be no physical reason? It is possible that your child was reminded of their past experience at the doctor's office and is experiencing hyperarousal. There is even a term for this: *white coat hypertension*.[3] This means that someone's blood pressure is higher when they come in to the doctor's office than when they are at home.[4] Thus, it is assumed that fears of the doctor or medical environment can affect blood pressure.

Our bodies can get stuck in a fight, flight, or freeze mode—even when the threat is gone.

When experiencing hyperarousal, sometimes children become jumpy. They may jump when a door opens or when someone walks into the room. They may have an elevated heart rate or blood pressure when a certain medical provider (or any medical provider) enters the room. They might have difficulty settling down to sleep or may wake up several times at night. These are signs of medical trauma.

AVOIDANCE

Avoidance can be a bit easier to recognize in children than the previous signs we've discussed. Symptoms of avoidance include trying not to think or talk about their medical condition or treatment or trying to avoid people, places, or things that remind them of their medical condition.

Does your child avoid talking about their medical condition or treatment? Do they get upset when they hear you talking about it? Do they try to refuse to go to medical appointments? Does it seem like your child is always running late when you're trying to leave for the doctor or the hospital? Does your child "have to go to the bathroom" when it's time to leave for an appointment or when a doctor walks in the room?

Children may act out before appointments in obvious ways. For example, they might refuse to get in the car or find other things to do, which makes them late. They may not even know why they are doing it. They may not be aware of their own fears.

Sometimes children avoid eye contact or interacting with medical team members. There can be many reasons for avoiding medications or treatments, but one reason is that treatment is a reminder of the medical condition. These are all possible signs of medical trauma.

CHILDREN WITH COMMUNICATION CHALLENGES

Although we'll go into more detail about the unique challenges of medical trauma in children with communication challenges or language barriers later in the book (chapter 28), it's important to note this here: it can be more difficult to recognize medical trauma symptoms in children who communicate differently or who have more difficulty communicating with us. If your child has communication challenges, it is helpful to watch their body responses and behaviors for patterns. Usually parents know their child best.

As a parent, you can look for the same behaviors or types of communication that you see when your child is unhappy or worried about other things. For example, when you give your child a snack that they do not like, what do they do? If you turn off their favorite TV show, how do they react? If they are afraid of the dark and their night light burns out, how do they normally respond?

Keeping your child's typical reactions in mind, observe how they act with medical providers, at the hospital, at the doctor's office, or during medical treatment. For example, does your child need extra support (such as nurses holding them) to be able to have their blood drawn or to have regular exams? If you see similar fearful or acting-out behaviors in the context of medical care, this could be a sign of medical trauma.

Other questions to ask yourself: Are your child's vitals elevated when they go for doctor's appointments? Does your child jump when someone opens a door to the clinic room? Is your child more oppositional when they know a medical appointment is coming? As a parent, you will likely be the first person to recognize that your child may be experiencing medical trauma, especially if your child has communication barriers.

None of these symptoms alone means that your child has medical trauma, but each of these are signs to watch for. Talk with your child's doctor if you have any concerns or questions about your child.

Medical Trauma in Cameron

Two months after Cameron's accident, he is still having nightmares. He tells his mom, Zoe, that sometimes he dreams about car accidents and other times about strange zombies. His dreams frequently involve the death of one of his parents. Each morning, it takes Cameron a very long time to get ready. Zoe helps him dress, since the casts and wheelchair make it hard for Cameron to dress himself. It often feels like she just can't get him moving. As a result, Cameron is regularly late to school and to his medical appointments.

Cameron's friends have been great about reaching out to him after the accident, but Cameron often skips activities with his friends. He prefers to be in his room when he is home, away from his family. This is different from how Cameron was before the accident: he used to love to hang with his friends as much as possible and enjoyed time with his family. Cameron has become quick to get angry with his brother and parents. When he rides in the car, he is often completely silent.

As a parent, you will likely be the first person to recognize your child's medical trauma.

His mom tries to talk to him about it, but he refuses. This starts to cause Zoe a lot of stress; she is worried about Cameron. Cameron and his brother, Emerson, are often late to school. Zoe is often late to work. She is starting to feel the stress that this situation has brought on the family. Preston, Cameron's dad, says not to worry about it, as he doesn't want to talk about the accident either. He says that he thinks it will all blow over in time.

After doing some research, Zoe begins to suspect that Cameron is experiencing medical trauma. Before the accident, Cameron was a carefree teenager; he only occasionally fought with his parents and was very close with his younger brother. While he has always liked to stay up late, he rarely had trouble sleeping or bad dreams prior to the accident.

Cameron's mother recognizes increased irritability, anger, and withdrawal in him. She also notices that he tries to avoid getting in the car. Zoe realizes that this might be why it is taking him so long to get ready to go places and why he sometimes misses out on activities with his friends.

Medical Trauma in Nia's Sibling

Earlier in this book, we met Nia when she was six months into treatment for cancer. Nia struggled with taking medications and cooperating with medical care. When Nia was first diagnosed with cancer, her mother, Maria, shifted her full focus onto taking care of her. Maria had always used a child-centered parenting approach. She gave Nia even more control when she learned Nia was sick. Maria didn't want to upset Nia. Maria wanted to give her daughter as much joy as possible.

Nia's older sister, Sara (age ten), also tried to help with Nia's treatment. Like her mother, she spent time trying to convince Nia to take her medications. Sara also gave up participating in her own activities to help with Nia and to try to make Nia happy.

At first, Sara showed no symptoms of medical trauma related to her sister's cancer and cancer treatment. She became extra cooperative with her mother, helping out even more than before. Sara never complained about her mother missing her activities or being at the hospital with Nia. She kept her grades up and stayed out of trouble. Sara never brought up Nia's cancer with anyone.

Maria isn't worried about Sara, because it seems like Sara is doing well. One evening though, at 11:00 p.m., Maria overhears Sara crying in her room. When Maria enters, Sara quickly stops crying and pretends that she is asleep. Later that week, Maria finds a journal that Sara had been writing in about how scared she is. Maria calls Sara's teacher to check in about how she is doing at school and learns that Sara has started to withdraw from her friends, spending time reading at recess rather than joining in activities.

Maria realizes that Sara has been putting on a brave face for the family but that she is experiencing medical trauma symptoms—lots of fear, problems sleeping, and starting to withdraw from her supportive friends.

Medical Trauma in Your Family

Cameron and Sara's symptoms are very common; they are often easy to recognize when we look back but very hard to see in the moment. We will learn a number of strategies that parents can use to help their children with these reactions in part 4 of the book.

Wondering if you or your child has medical trauma? Take a look at the checklist below. If you think you as a caregiver might suffer from medical trauma, you can consider this list, but be sure to find the checklist especially designed for you in chapter 30.

MEDICAL TRAUMA CHECKLIST

This checklist provides a list of possible symptoms of medical trauma that children may experience. It is not a replacement for having your child evaluated by a professional if you are concerned. If your child (or child's siblings) experience any of the symptoms below, it could be a sign of medical trauma. Talk with your child's doctor about any of your concerns. Share this checklist with your doctor to help them understand your concerns.

My child

_____ talks a lot about their medical condition or medical care
_____ refuses to talk about their condition or medical care
_____ gets upset when talking about their condition or medical care
_____ has dreams about their condition or medical care
_____ has bad dreams or nightmares
_____ has strong body reactions (e.g., racing heart, fast breathing, stomachache) when they think or talk about their condition or medical care
_____ feels mad a lot
_____ feels sad a lot
_____ feels bad a lot
_____ worries a lot
_____ is really jumpy
_____ has trouble sleeping
_____ has trouble paying attention
_____ makes us late to medical appointments

QUESTIONS TO ASK YOURSELF

- How has my child's medical journey changed our family?
- Does anyone in my family show signs of medical trauma?

ACTION STEPS

- Complete the checklist with your child or for your child. Make notes of any symptoms in your C.O.A.C.H. notebook that you want to share with your child's doctor.
- Complete the checklist with or for your child's siblings. Make notes of any symptoms in your C.O.A.C.H. notebook that you want to share with your child's doctor.

6

What *Isn't* Medical Trauma?

Not great, Mommy. Poopy. Butt cheeks.

—A four-year-old child's response to how he was feeling after a stomach surgery

Figuring out why kids act the way they do can be difficult, especially in stressful situations such as medical appointments or procedures. With children who are undergoing significant medical treatment or who have suddenly become terrified of their pediatrician's office, it can be even trickier.

Young children can also be challenging to understand: in the quote above, it is tough to know what "not great" means. Is the child in pain? Or afraid? Or bored? Understanding what is causing a child's behaviors or emotions can be important in deciding what strategies to try to help them manage their reactions.

In the previous chapter, we described medical trauma reactions as changes in mood, reexperiencing, hyperarousal, and avoidance. This can cover a lot of behaviors and emotions, but it is also important not to overlook other emotional health challenges while navigating your child's medical journey.

Some common challenges that could be part of medical trauma or might stand on their own include

- ongoing pain,
- oppositional behaviors,
- attention deficit hyperactivity disorder,
- anxiety,
- depression,
- other traumas (e.g., experiencing abuse in their past or witnessing violence), and
- sleep problems.

There are some hints to determine whether a particular behavior or symptom might *not* be medical trauma or might be medical trauma *plus* other challenges. Think back to before your child had a medical condition or injury (if there was such a time) or before your child became frightened of medical appointments. If the behaviors started before the medical condition or fear, then they likely are not caused solely by your child's medical experience.

For example, if your child had a lot of separation anxiety as a young child and now is having trouble sleeping as an eight-year-old, they may have anxiety that preexisted their medical condition. If your child has always been strong-willed and struggled with following rules and is now having trouble following directions related to their medical care, there may be other emotional health challenges to consider, such as attention deficit hyperactivity disorder or oppositional defiant disorder.

In learning about your child's medical condition, you may also learn that there are certain behaviors or emotions that are common to their condition. For example, children with autism are often sensitive to touch or sounds, regardless of the reason (whether medical or not).

Another hint could be your family's health history. If any of your child's biological relatives had attention deficit hyperactivity disorder, oppositional behaviors, anxiety, depression, or other emotional health conditions, it may be that your child is experiencing these symptoms independent of their medical experiences.

Pain can be particularly tricky to figure out in children. Uncontrolled pain, whether ongoing or sporadic, can make it more likely that your child will develop medical trauma. It also can cause challenging behaviors on its own. To start to identify how pain might be affecting your child, it may be helpful to write down things that you see your child doing when you suspect or know they have pain. Are they more irritable? More tired? More down? Do they sleep more? Do they have more sleep problems?

If you are trying to figure out if your child's behaviors might be related to pain or have other causes, try tracking their pain and worrisome behaviors. Write down times when you know your child is in pain, along with how your child behaves during these times. Write down times when you observe your child's concerning behaviors. By tracking your child's pain, attempts at pain control, and behaviors together, you may be able to work with your child's medical team to figure out what is causing your child's challenging behaviors (pain versus medical trauma or other emotional health challenges).

We also can't ignore the possibility of other traumas in your child's life. As we noted in the previous chapter, other traumas make the development of medical trauma more likely. Other traumas also can exist on their own, outside of medically related trauma. Experiences such as physical, sexual, or psychological abuse; neglect; family or community violence; sudden or violent loss of a loved one; a personal or family member's substance use disorder; refugee or war experiences; and military family–related stressors (e.g., deployment, parental loss or injury) are all recognized as potential sources of trauma in children, in addition to medical events. In the United States, 60 percent of children and adolescents have experienced or witnessed a potentially traumatic event.[1]

Consider the possibility of other traumas in your child's life.

If your child is having reactions that are creating a lot of stress in your family, that interfere with their medical care, with school, or with other activities they want to do, talk with your child's doctor to learn where to get more help.

Daniel: It's Not Only Medical Trauma

When we met Daniel, we learned that he has Hunter syndrome. Hunter syndrome can include emotional health symptoms similar to those of autism spectrum disorders, attention deficit hyperactivity disorder, and sensory processing disorder. Daniel's grandparents think that they recognize some medical trauma symptoms as his anxiety increases at each hospital appointment. They also consider how some of his behaviors could be associated with Hunter syndrome. As mentioned earlier in this book (see chapter 2), Daniel's anxiety in getting ready for medical appointments and his response "no, no, no" are likely related to his medical experiences.

However, some of his anxiety may also be linked to communication challenges that are a part of autism spectrum disorder and his tendency to become overstimulated (part of autism spectrum disorder and sensory processing disorder). For example, with limited communication, he may not be able to understand exactly what to expect at his doctor's appointments. In addition, sensory challenges may make Daniel experience seemingly pain-free procedures and exams as uncomfortable or even painful. Something as simple as a doctor using a stethoscope to listen to their breathing or heart rate can be uncomfortable for people with sensory challenges.

While some of Daniel's reactions may be part of Hunter syndrome, medical trauma can also add challenges. For example, if Daniel has negative experiences with an exam, then future exams may become emotionally traumatic for him. More specifically, if Daniel has to be held down or has many people yelling at him to calm down or be still, this could set the stage for future appointments. Each time he needs another exam, he may have reexperiencing or hyperarousal symptoms.

Daniel's grandparents are able to describe his challenges to his doctors in the course of his regular appointments. Together, the medical team and his grandparents are able to sort out which of Daniel's reactions are likely related to medical trauma, which are related to Hunter syndrome, and which might be related to both. Daniel's medical team is then able to provide guidance and treatment related to typical Hunter syndrome behaviors, while his grandparents work with his medical team on strategies to minimize his medical trauma.

QUESTIONS TO ASK YOURSELF

- How long have my child's challenging behaviors been happening?
- Did I or my child's other parent do anything like this when we were younger?

ACTION STEPS

- Observe your child's behaviors. In your C.O.A.C.H. notebook, write down these behaviors. Make notes of what time it is and what other things are happening in the room when your child is showing challenging behaviors.
- In your C.O.A.C.H. notebook, track your child's pain and what you are doing to manage it.
- Make a list of questions to share with your child's medical team.

7

Medical Sprints versus Medical Marathons

I have to see marathons in fifty-yard dashes.

—Davita Hungate, trauma survivor

Running a one-hundred-yard dash is quite different than running a 26.2-mile marathon. Sprinting requires an explosion of energy, but the effort is only required for a short time. At the end, the sprinter is breathing heavily but then can rest and recover. Marathoners, on the other hand, have to pace themselves. They have to maintain psychological and physical balance over a long period of time. They have to reserve enough energy to continue the race mile after mile. They may get leg cramps, blisters, or other aches that come with sustaining activity for long periods of time.

The training for sprints is also different than for distance running. The equipment varies as well—sprinting shoes are not marathon shoes. It's all running, but sprints are not marathons and marathons are not sprints.

Luckily for runners, they know ahead of time the type of race they are running. They can choose how to train, their equipment, and their psychological preparation. They run the practice race many times before the one that counts.

When it comes to a medical challenge, sometimes we know whether the challenge is a sprint (e.g., helping a child through a vaccine) or a marathon (e.g., helping a child through treatment for cancer or a lifelong genetic condition). Other times, the twists and turns of the medical condition are completely unpredictable. Sprints can turn into marathons. Sometimes we may need to sprint within a marathon. For example, your child might need a short hospitalization for an infection or to receive a particular medication. This may be a sprint for you and your family. You may need to juggle a few things around, but you get prepared for this short treatment. Then you find out the medication didn't work. Your child ends up in the hospital for weeks and then months, changing what seemed like a sprint into a marathon.

> *You can run a sprint or you can run a marathon, but you can't sprint a marathon.*
>
> —*Ryan Holmes*

If only we all knew ahead of time what our child's journey would look like, we could better prepare ourselves. If only we knew that the broken leg would result in further surgeries and years of physical therapy, that those seemingly unrelated symptoms would turn into a diagnosable genetic condition, that we would continue to search for a diagnosis for years without ever finding one, or that the illness is completely treatable and we just have to power through for a short time.

Unfortunately, we often don't know whether part of our child's medical journey will turn into a marathon or when. And sometimes, by the time we realize it is indeed a marathon, we've been sprinting about ten miles and we're exhausted—physically, mentally, emotionally, spiritually. As Canadian businessman Ryan Holmes put it, "You can run a sprint or you can run a marathon, but you can't sprint a marathon."

So how do we find balance when we can't see the future? How do our strategies for preventing and managing medical trauma differ when we consider medical sprints versus medical marathons?

If we're looking at a sprint, such as some upcoming challenging doctor's appointments or a surgery, or even in some cases a cancer diagnosis, we can often run fast, even full speed if necessary, for a period of time. Depending on the seriousness of the medical challenge, our child's care can become top priority, and everything else can be put on hold.

If you believe you're in a medical sprint, these tips may be helpful:

- Stay calm. Your child takes their cues from you.
- Write things down. Many parents find that when they've been sprinting, it can help to have notes to refer to or to share among caregivers and with medical team members.
- Check in regularly with your child. Check to see if your child understands what is going on (if they are able to), what to expect next, and who will be there to support them.

Whether it's a sprint or a marathon, one key is to look at your child's medical challenges in the context of their whole life, not just their *medical* life. It's tempting to compartmentalize our child's medical life as separate from their *real* life. Many times we think, if we can just get past *this* medical hurdle, we can get back to *real* life.

But here is what we know. All the other aspects of your child's life affect how they respond to medical interventions. And medical trauma responses can affect many other areas of your child's life. In the end, there is no *medical life* or *real life*; it is just *their life.*

Thinking in terms of marathons: looking ahead, you may be able to anticipate particular medical challenges as uphills or downhills, some harder and some easier. As we know with all parenting, there will be surprises mixed in. There will likely be both good and bad surprises. No matter what is put in front of us in our child's medical journey, we can learn to adjust the same way we adjusted to other parts of parenting—toddlerhood, school transitions, teen rebellion.

With that being said, there are some strategies that can help us run those medical marathons that may be more uphill than downhill.

PACE YOURSELF

When your child is suddenly injured or receives a new diagnosis, one of the most difficult things to do as a parent is to pace yourself. You may feel like you've been hit by a ton of bricks. Different parents respond in different ways. For some parents, it's tempting to drop everything. Jump in the deep end. Learn as much as possible. Take action. For others, everything may seem so overwhelming that you freeze and have a hard time making decisions. Both of these reactions are normal.

Uday Kotak, an Indian billionaire banker, had it right when he said, "In a marathon, if you run too fast, you get exhausted. If you run too slow, you never make it." In other words, pace yourself.

If you tend to jump in and spend all day reading about your child's diagnosis and talking to experts or other parents of similar children, at some point you will burn out. Slow your sprinting down.

If you are frozen on the spot and can't seem to process what is going on with your child, take one step at a time. Ask one question. Take notes. Just keep moving.

Self-care helps you maintain the mental, emotional, and physical reserves to support your child over the long run. What that looks like can be different for everyone.

ASSEMBLE YOUR WATER TEAM

If you've ever run a race, you know how good it feels to have people encouraging you on the sidelines. You may need encouragement at the beginning, in the middle as you're getting tired, and at the end. Having people who are both emotionally supporting you and also tangibly providing you with what you need to keep going is essential. That is your water team, also known as your support system.

Self-care helps you maintain the mental, emotional, and physical reserves to support your child over the long run.

As we mentioned in earlier chapters, identify your support team and let them know how important their role is. Sometimes you might need someone to carry you through part of the journey.

TAKE A BREAK

Parenting a child without medical challenges is hard enough.

If you consider that your child's medical journey is a marathon, you will need a break. This is not selfish. This is necessary.

Breaks will look different for different parents. For some, it might look like ten minutes away from their child to call a friend. Others may take an hour for lunch or a walk. For some, a weekend away is needed. Some parents also find spending time at work to be a break from caregiving. What matters most is that you take the time for yourself and come back feeling a bit more refreshed than when you left. This gives you energy for the marathon that may be ahead of you.

Your well-being is a key part of helping your child. Filling your own tank allows you to continue to provide the best support possible.

Ask someone in your support system to make sure you take breaks. They may even be able to help you with the logistics of taking time away, such as staying with your child or helping you find someone who will.

Cameron: Sprinting into a Marathon

After Cameron's car accident, his parents hoped that life would soon get back to normal. They wished that Cameron's legs would heal quickly so they could kiss the hospital goodbye. But surgeries and rehab lasted a lot longer than they anticipated.

At first, Cameron's mom, Zoe, thought they could put regular life on hold, get Cameron well, then go back to life as they knew it. But every week brings more changes. The surgeries are stressful. They have to juggle who takes Cameron to appointments, who communicates with his teachers, and who encourages him to do his exercises.

In the midst of Cameron's medical challenges, they also can't forget about Emerson's needs. It helps that he stayed with his grandparents during the really demanding period right after the accident, while Cameron had several surgeries, but now Cameron is home, and things still aren't the same. Emerson is feeling lonely without Cameron to interact with like usual. As for his parents, Zoe and Preston are often preoccupied with Cameron's medical needs. Preston is particularly concerned that Cameron will never walk again.

Your well-being is a key part of helping your child.

Cameron himself grows more withdrawn and agitated as time goes on. He tells his mom and doctors that he didn't realize his recovery would take so long.

A few weeks after the surgeries, a physical therapist at the hospital recognizes Cameron's anxiety and that his expectations of his recovery process are unrealistic. Working with his doctor, the medical team has a discussion with Cameron and his parents about what the next several months might look like. They talk about how Cameron should celebrate some milestones to help him feel like he is making progress. Having more realistic expectations also helps Zoe and Preston stop holding their breath when it comes to making changes to help their family function during Cameron's recovery.

Jin: What Kind of Race Are We Running?

When Jin first struggled with vaccinations, her parents assumed her fear was like that of many other children when it came to getting their shots. They comforted her, got through it, and didn't think much about it. Then, when she struggled so much in the emergency room and with other medical appointments, they realized this might be a bigger problem than they had thought.

Now that Jin is facing daily finger sticks, insulin shots, and possibly an insulin pump, Amy and Cole are worried about how to explain everything to her given her communication challenges. They worry that Jin will start hating them. But they have to make sure her diabetes is well controlled.

Once Jin's parents understand that she is likely experiencing medical trauma, they start to learn how to help her. They go with Jin to see a pediatric psychologist at the children's hospital. The pediatric psychologist asks them questions about Jin's medical care and her responses. The psychologist also observes her during a medical appointment. Working with the psychologist, Jin's parents are able to identify what parts of medical care are the hardest for her. They look forward to working with the psychologist to learn some strategies they can use to support Jin in monitoring and treating her diabetes as well as before and during her medical appointments. They hope that, over time, they can help her feel more relaxed and comfortable with the medical treatments and appointments that she will need.

QUESTIONS TO ASK YOURSELF

- Which medical challenges in my child's life could be described as sprints? As marathons?
- Are there events in my life that I thought would be sprints but became marathons?

- Who in my support system helps me with day-to-day survival (e.g., managing doctor's appointments, caring for my children, grocery shopping, picking up medications)?
- Who in my support system do I turn to for support as a parent (e.g., ask for ideas when my child is showing difficult behaviors; ask for support when I feel overwhelmed, afraid, or sad)?

ACTION STEPS

- Identify ways in which you've treated your child's journey as a sprint (e.g., put things off, not taken time for self-care).
- In your C.O.A.C.H. notebook, write down the one thing that you will do for yourself to help pace yourself over the course of your child's medical journey.
- Ask someone in your support system to help you schedule a break within the next month—a coffee break, an evening alone, a Saturday with friends, whatever sounds right to you.

8

Your Family and the Health Care System

You treat a disease, you win, you lose. You treat a person, I guarantee you, you'll win, no matter what the outcome.

—Hunter "Patch" Adams, played by
Robin Williams in the movie *Patch Adams*

Medical appointments and procedures don't exist in a vacuum. Gone are the days of house calls where one doctor treats your whole family. Instead, what we often see is a complex network of doctors, administrators, nurses, and specialists. You're not just dealing with one health care provider but an entire system. This modern health care model can bring both advantages and additional challenges.

It helps to take a step back and look at all the interactions your child has had with the health care system in the past as well as the interactions your child might have in the future. Does your child go to a teaching hospital where medical students pop into the room to hear about your child's condition? Does your child have a great team of experts who work well together? Does their pediatrician vary, depending on who is available? Are there long waits when they go to see a specialist?

A shift has occurred in recent years toward providing family-focused care for children (i.e., considering how medical care/

conditions affect the whole family). We now know that family-centered care can improve the quality of care provided.[1] Another shift is increased access to medical specialists and interdisciplinary teams for treating children. However, there remain aspects of the health care system's structure that may make it harder for you to prevent, identify, and/or manage your child's medical trauma. Some of these features include a history of paternalism (doctor knows best), care silos (lack of coordination among doctors/specialists), and reactionary medicine (treating a condition and its symptoms after it develops instead of preventing it).

Let's take a look at the most common historical challenges and some strategies you can use to navigate them for the benefit of your child.

A HISTORY OF "DOCTOR KNOWS BEST"

We've all heard the phrase "doctor knows best," and for you, it might evoke positive, neutral, or negative feelings. Historically in medicine, that concept was known as paternalism. It operated as doctors acting to promote their patients' good or prevent their harm, which sounds good in theory:

> For at least 2,500 years, the doctor-patient relationship has resembled the parent-child relationship. The norms of medical ethics . . . encouraged doctors to shield patients from bad news and from general medical knowledge. While Western medical tradition has always included some patient protections, such as informed consent (and its antecedents), doctors have possessed broad powers to withhold treatments that patients desired and, at times, to mislead patients for what they perceived to be the patients' own good.[2]

Forms of paternalism can help protect us in many areas of our life. For example, experts have learned that seat belts and helmets can prevent injuries and have advocated for laws to force us to follow these rules. Even in medicine, we must be able to depend on doctors' recommendations, since many of us may not understand the complexities of a medical condition. It's not uncommon that we prefer to defer to the medical team and let them recommend the best course for ourselves or our children; that is a choice we can make.

But problems can emerge if a philosophy of "doctor knows best" trumps specific preferences of families regarding their child's care.

Medical decision making generally requires informed consent, which means that health care providers must explain the nature and purpose of a proposed procedure. This includes the potential burdens, benefits, and risks related to that procedure. This also includes alternative treatments so that patients or their caregivers have all the relevant information to decide whether or not to proceed.[3]

While medical providers are required to obtain permission from parents and often work to include children and parents in both short-term and long-term planning for medical care, this doesn't always work as intended. At times, discussions between medical providers and families are led by providers who may have very strong opinions about what is best for their patient. Strong opinions from medical providers can overwhelm vulnerable patients and their families. In addition, sometimes medical teams think that certain information has been communicated to parents, but it may have slipped through the cracks.

Informed consent means that health care providers must explain the nature and purpose of a proposed procedure.

In its most positive light, paternalism tries to account for the fact that patients and caregivers don't have a medical education and may not fully appreciate the medical issues involved. Medical providers usually care deeply for the children they are treating and want to be sure the treatment is the best possible for the child and family. Sometimes this comes out as providers directing parents and children on what to do.

In its most negative light, paternalism can result in a medical team not listening to a child and/or the child's family. It can result in the medical team deciding instead that they know what is best for the child and being unwilling to consider other options or continue to discuss questions with a family.

In recent years, there has been a huge shift to provide family-centered care, which centers around communicating with the family and ensuring families are involved in medical planning and decision making. As appreciation has grown for considering patient and family perspectives, needs, and opinions, fewer medical providers are taking a hard stance of "I know what's best for your child." Increased accessibility to reliable medical information has also helped to create a more well-informed and empowered patient population.[4]

Most medical professionals respect the concerns of parents and caregivers. But it can be helpful to be aware of the history of medicine as you advocate for your child's needs. The challenge of medical trauma is not yet well known, sometimes even in the medical community. Some of your child's medical professionals might not know how to best guide you if you are concerned about medical trauma in your child. If, in order to accommodate your child's needs, you make suggestions for how things should proceed with appointments or request that medical professionals modify their style, that medical professional might believe that their plan works better. Communicating with your medical team is essential to getting the best care for your child.

CARE SILOS

When most medical care was carried out by family doctors, the doctor knew and treated the whole patient. They likely knew their patient's whole family and family history. With the advancement of medicine, specializations multiplied. Medical specialization has improved health care for many children with chronic health conditions, but challenges in communicating about children's care also grew.

Thankfully, the system has been changing over the years, much to the benefit of patients and their families. Collaborative medical approaches, electronic medical records, and the power of informed patients have driven medical care toward a more patient-centric approach. This can benefit patients' overall health.

Even so, sometimes it can be quite frustrating when medical teams or specialists are not communicating with one another. How well your medical teams work together can depend on your health system, your location, and individual providers.

To help advocate for consistent care for your child, there are several steps you can take to break down the obstacles posed by medical care silos, including staying organized, seeking care within one medical system, and maintaining a summary of your child's health challenges in their medical records. Consider creating a written document to share with all medical team members. This can help you remember all the important information and have something to share so you do not have to repeat yourself to different providers as frequently.

REACTIONARY MEDICINE

In the past, medicine focused on managing symptoms and dealing with illnesses, injuries, or diseases as they emerged—for example, treating heart attacks or injuries from car crashes.

Only recently has medicine shifted to include prevention, wellness visits, and screenings. This new focus helps to prevent diseases or injuries and catch problems early. For example, pediatricians now evaluate children's eating and nutrition and encourage safety behaviors such as wearing a seat belt. Doctors now also monitor and prescribe medications in order to help prevent heart attacks.

In the past, medical trauma and emotional distress may have been overlooked until they got really bad—for example, when a child's fighting out of fear prevented them from getting a life-saving medication. But now we can build on the growing importance of preventative medicine.

Medical trauma can be regularly assessed and managed early on. Regular screening can help you and your child's medical team identify early symptoms of medical trauma. While there is a growing understanding and awareness of medical trauma within the medical community, not all medical providers know exactly what it means. One great resource for medical providers and parents to learn more about medical trauma is www.HealthCareToolbox.org.

WHAT DOES THIS MEAN FOR MEDICAL TRAUMA AND YOUR CHILD?

Although the challenges of paternalism, care silos, and reactionary medicine still exist in health care, they are declining. The opportunities for you as a parent to prevent and manage medical trauma in your child are greater than ever.

Let's look at how the health care system affects patients, using the patient stories we've followed in this book.

Daniel and the Overwhelming Diagnosis

When Daniel's mother, Sandy, first brought him to the geneticist at almost three years old, she wasn't sure why they were there. Daniel's pediatrician had said something about "coarse facial features" and a large belly, but to Sandy he just looked like any cute little boy.

At their next visit with the geneticist, Sandy hoped to learn if there was anything wrong with her little guy.

The doctor entered the office with a specialist who introduced herself as a genetic counselor. Then the doctor started talking about this really long name of a disease (mucopolysaccharidosis II) and told Sandy *not* to go home and search for it on the Internet. He said that the genetic counselor would be getting in touch with her to start scheduling appointments. He asked if she had any questions, but Sandy didn't even understand enough to have questions. She took the printouts he gave her and left in a daze. Her son looked healthy, but now she was realizing he wasn't. She didn't know what that would mean for Daniel or for her.

The next week, she got a call from the genetic counselor, who set up several appointments for Daniel. Cardiology, orthopaedics, neurology, audiology, pulmonology—the list went on and on. Then the counselor said that Daniel would need to be scheduled for surgery to get a port-a-cath placed to receive a weekly infusion of medicine. It was more than Sandy could take. She didn't feel like she could manage this. She asked her parents for help.

After several long and heart-rending discussions with Sandy, Daniel's grandparents agreed to take charge of his medical care. They took over as his primary caretakers. They brought him to his next appointment with the geneticist a few weeks later. By this time, they had done some research about possible medications and clinical trials that might help Daniel. A clinical trial involves research where physicians use new and promising but unproven medicines with the goal of seeing if the medicines are effective to treat a condition. Nana and Papa had read that there were some new potential treatments for Hunter syndrome in clinical trials. They had a lot of questions for the geneticist and the genetic counselor.

Nana and Papa asked what the team knew about the clinical trials they read about. They also asked whether they could schedule Daniel's appointments in a way that made sense for him. They preferred not to do the appointments all in one day because it was too overwhelming for Daniel. They asked about how to have easy access to Daniel's medical records after he saw all these doctors and who would be the person in charge of Daniel's care. This time, with his grandparents advocating for him, Daniel's geneticist took care to listen to the family's ideas and needs for Daniel.

QUESTIONS TO ASK YOURSELF

- Has a medical provider ever not listened or minimized my concerns about my child? How did I address it?
- How do my child's medical providers communicate with one another, and how are the medical records coordinated?
- What are some ways that preventative medicine helps my child, and how might that apply in the case of medical trauma?

ACTION STEPS

- In your C.O.A.C.H. notebook, write down your child's medical challenges, including their medical trauma reactions and any triggers you can identify.
- As you read through the rest of this book, note the strategies that you think would help your child in future medical events.
- If needed, figure out the best time to speak with your child's medical provider(s) about the issue of medical trauma (e.g., at the beginning of the next medical appointment, via a phone call, through an online portal).

Part 3

WHO ARE YOU?

9

You Are a Person, Then a Parent

What we know matters, but who we are matters more.

—Brené Brown, *Daring Greatly: How the Courage to Be Vulnerable Transforms the Way We Live, Love, Parent, and Lead*

When Amy's daughter, Jin, was first diagnosed with type 1 diabetes, Amy joined an online support group of local parents of children with diabetes. The group helped her find a local doctor, learn what her school system usually did to accommodate her child's medical needs, and find information about medical suppliers in the area. Even as she talked more with people in the group about things outside of diabetes, she still thought of them as her "diabetes friends." She didn't consider them "real" friends.

After multiple crises in her daughter's care, however, Amy slowly learned more about some of her diabetes friends, and they learned more about her outside of the context of their children's condition. At one point, it felt like her worlds were colliding. She couldn't decide whether that was a good thing or a bad thing.

After Jin was diagnosed with diabetes, Amy also had trouble juggling all her different roles and expectations. To the diabetes support group, she was the parent of a child with type 1 diabetes with certain challenges and particular needs. But to her other friends, she was

Amy, a fun friend who always told the best stories and was there with a listening ear. To her kids, she was a parent. To her colleagues, she was a human resources director. To her daughter's class, she was the homeroom mom.

In this section, we'll discuss the roles that can be important when parenting a child through medical trauma. While we discuss the strengths, challenges, and strategies in each role, you may want to consider how each role fits into your full person. Just as viewing your child's medical experiences as part of their life can help in parenting through medical challenges, understanding your own roles and expectations can help you decide how to manage things.

YOU AS A PERSON

This section of the book asks the question, "Who are you?" You can start by asking yourself, "Who am I?" Then ask yourself how people in your life would describe you. For example, how would your children, your work colleagues, or your friends describe you?

There's no wrong answer.

In decades past, our families and communities were physically closer and more interdependent. Our identity was formed more from the roles and beliefs of our parents and what the community expected of us. As society has shifted away from interwoven communities, we have more individual choice about our identity. When we become a parent of a child with a medical condition or other challenges, our identity may shift or change.

Our identity has many layers, and it develops in a lifelong process as our needs, desires, experiences, and environments change. Generally, it can be said that our identity is a function of the following layers:

- **Facts:** factual characteristics such as your height, ethnicity, where you live, your income level, and your marital status
- **Actions:** our choices in what we do and how we shape our life (e.g., I read bedtime stories to my kids, I became a nurse)
- **Cares:** what we care about tends to be reflected in our actions, but we can engage in the same action for different reasons

- **Beliefs:** what we believe in forms the narrative of our life story and is also reflected in our actions, such as who and what you affiliate with, where you donate, and what you read or watch
- **Values:** what we value in life can also drive our beliefs, cares, and actions, such as valuing time with others or monetary success

Our identity has many layers, and it develops in a lifelong process as our needs, desires, experiences, and environments change.

As parenting begins, it is common for parents to lose sight of and/or time for many of our own interests, hobbies, and opinions. Sometimes we get caught up in the important roles we play in raising our children. This can be magnified when parenting a child with a medical condition.

YOU AS A PARENT

According to the Pew Research Center report "Parenting in America," 94 percent of parents said that their role as a parent is very or extremely important to their identity.[1] If you're reading this book, chances are that you take your role as a parent seriously and you invest time and energy into your parenting.

As we touched on in chapter 2, how you normally parent your child will typically affect how you will parent them through medical challenges. In walking with your child on their medical journey, you will likely have many experiences of supporting your child through medical challenges, helping them manage their reactions, and caring for them. While supporting your child, you are also experiencing their medical events in your own capacity as a person, which means that you could also develop medical trauma related to your child's medical condition and/or treatment (see chapter 30 for more information on this).

While most parents believe they're doing at least a good job at parenting overall, one-third of parents note that they feel rushed all the time and that they spend too little time with their children.[2] As we'll discuss later in the book, preventing and managing medical trauma in your child or in yourself often involves thinking ahead and putting new systems into place. This can be challenging if you're already rushed and disconnected. If that's the case, everything associated with coping with your child's medical challenge may sound overwhelming right now.

This book offers a range of strategies for you to try, building on what you already know, one step at a time. Keep in mind that you know your child and your family best. You can choose what to take from this book and what to leave.

So how do you balance fulfilling your typical responsibilities as a parent with supporting your child in their medical needs and with potential medical trauma? Here are a few ideas to remember:

- **Time:** Take your time. You don't need to integrate what you learn from this book all at once.
- **Working with your child:** It is most helpful to involve your child, either when choosing strategies (if they are able) or in thinking about what you know about your child and yourself and choosing what might work best for your family.
- **Trial and error:** Not all strategies work for all kids and families. If you give one a try and it doesn't work, move on to the next. Discovering that something doesn't work for you or your child is learning, not failure.

We'll touch on these ideas more in the next few chapters and suggest small changes you can start trying out. Your role as a parent will help support your child through these challenges.

(Grand)Parenting Daniel

Daniel's grandparents were empty nesters when their daughter Sandy first called to tell them she was pregnant. They could tell she was nervous about how she would manage her job and support a child on her own. Nana and Papa wanted to help, but they also had just retired and started traveling and enjoying their freedom.

They offered to help watch the baby after Daniel was born while Sandy worked. They continued activities they enjoyed, like walks in the park and bingo at church. They just brought little Daniel with them. This partnership worked well for several years. Sandy was able to work, and Nana and Papa got to spend lots of time with their precious grandson.

As a toddler, Daniel experienced some medical challenges, including a surgery to repair a hernia he was born with. He seemed to take the medical appointments and surgeries in stride. Nana and Papa tried to support Sandy as much as they could, especially during these medical challenges. Although they were helping out with Daniel a lot, Nana and Papa still enjoyed a full life without parenting responsibilities. However, after Daniel's diagnosis and Sandy's decision to ask them to raise Daniel, they had to make a lot of changes.

As they transitioned from their role as grandparents to their new role as primary guardians of Daniel, they started cutting back on their own activities. With Daniel's new diagnosis of Hunter syndrome, there were so many more doctor's appointments and hospital visits. And, being in their late sixties, they were very tired by the end of the day. They could feel themselves getting frustrated at starting over as parents and at their involvement in a medical system that felt overwhelming at times.

As Daniel's needs continued to grow, Nana and Papa decided they had to balance Daniel's medical life with the joy and activities they had looked forward to before taking on full-time care for Daniel. They started planning fun activities and short trips surrounding Daniel's weekly hospital visits for infusions. They found places they always wanted to visit so that they could enjoy their travels once again while still caring for Daniel.

QUESTIONS TO ASK YOURSELF

- How would I describe myself and the roles that I am juggling?
- Do my actions reflect what I consider to be my cares, beliefs, and values?
- What do I do on a regular basis to care for myself?
- How do I balance being my own person with being a parent?

ACTION STEPS

- In your C.O.A.C.H. notebook, make a list of your current roles. Place a star next to your most important roles.
- Pick a part of your identity that you really love or that is really important to you. List three things you can do to grow that part of you.

10

You Are a Caregiver

> I belong to the people I love, and they belong to me—they, and the love and loyalty I give them, form my identity far more than any word or group ever could.
>
> —Veronica Roth, *Allegiant*

Many of us feel an intense love and instinct to care for our child from the first moment they enter our family, whether by birth or adoption. For birth parents, these instincts can start much earlier as the baby's first kicks and demands are felt during pregnancy. During our child's early years, we grow into our new role as caregiver as we feed them and change diapers, rock them to sleep, and calm their cries (or spend hours trying!). We learn about how to meet their needs better and about what they like and don't like. We can spend hours thinking about their health and safety.

In other words, we become their caregiver, in many forms of the word, from the moment they are ours.

Being a caregiver often becomes part of our identity early on as a parent. The role of parent can sometimes feel synonymous with caregiver, especially for the primary caregiver. However, they are distinct. As our children age, we remain their parent forever (although that role changes as well). With typically developing children, our caregiving lessens over time as our children grow into adults. If we have children with special health care needs, our caregiving role can remain constant even as they age. In the case of neurodegenerative conditions, caregiving often increases as the severity of our child's condition increases.

When our children are young, caregiving is both emotional and functional. On one hand, the emotional aspect of caregiving includes our love for them. We develop emotional and psychological attachments to our children that help them feel cared for and learn how relationships work at a basic level. On the functional level, we provide for their physical and tangible needs—food, clothing, a bed, supervision, and safety.

The emotional and functional roles of caregiving can also be described as nurturing. You are nurturing your child—encouraging their growth and development in becoming a person separate from you.

Caregiving in the context of your child's medical challenges falls somewhere in between emotional and functional caregiving. In the case of caring for a child with a chronic condition, it has been described as mothering plus extras.[1] Whatever your child's medical challenge, be it short term, long term, life-threatening, or mildly problematic, caregiving in the context of medical needs can sometimes feel less like being a nurturer and more like being an unpaid medical or care provider.

For example, we've met Cameron in earlier chapters. Cameron was thirteen years old when he was in a car crash that resulted in serious injuries. Prior to his injuries, his parents were slowly giving him more freedom and responsibility, as one would expect with a typical thirteen-year-old. Both of his parents' roles as caregivers were changing. Cameron no longer needed his parents' help with most of his activities of daily living. The functional caregiving role of his parents had been decreasing as he became more independent. Of course, his parents still made many of the meals and transported Cameron to activities and to meet friends. But he could now choose his own clothes, manage his schoolwork, and take care of his sports schedules.

Even on the emotional side, Cameron began to depend increasingly on his friends for support. In previous years, his parents and siblings had provided the majority of Cameron's emotional caregiving.

But once Cameron was injured, he turned to his mother, Zoe, for that unique caregiving role that relates to medical challenges. Zoe learned about all his injuries and necessary rehab, taught Cameron what she learned, and took on the task of monitoring Cameron's condition.

Over time, Cameron will again be able to take on some of the responsibilities that his mother assumed. But we see in the context of medical care a unique addition to the caregiver role.

It is not uncommon for caregivers of children with medical needs to feel distress over the change in caregiving responsibilities, especially if a child's needs are long term or chronic. For many parents, caring for a child with a chronic health condition is oftentimes accompanied by feelings of sadness and grief and a sense of being overwhelmed.[2] Parents often look to gain a sense of control in how to manage their child's condition and can become hypervigilant, monitoring symptoms and medical needs because they feel responsible for their child's health.

It is not uncommon for caregivers of children with medical needs to feel distress over the change in caregiving responsibilities, especially if a child's needs are long term or chronic.

If your child has experienced a sudden medical change, as in Cameron's case, it can be hard to shift caregiving responsibilities within your family or community. Other children and families in your social circle might have different freedoms than your family. Your family's routine may be more limited either temporarily or more permanently due to your child's medical condition. This can make maintaining your own identity more challenging.

The responsibilities in caring for our children change and shift over time, ebbing and flowing, sometimes slowly and sometimes in an instant with an unexpected diagnosis. Understanding our identity—first as our own person, then as a parent, and then as a caregiver—helps us manage sometimes overwhelming feelings that can accompany a shift in what our role as a caregiver might demand.

In the next chapter, we'll talk about how in your role as a caregiver you can interact with your child's medical providers to become a leader of your child's medical team.

Maria's Shifting Role as Nia's Caregiver

When her daughters were toddlers, Maria loved to teach them new things. She made potty training fun with M&M rewards and princess potties. She made flashcards for letters when they were learning their ABCs. The three of them would learn funny dances to the latest music and practice together. One of her tricks was to make certain chores into rewards. The girls would *get to* unload the dishwasher or vacuum the floor if they were good.

Slowly, as all children do, the girls started becoming more independent. They liked to pick out their own clothes and got wise to Maria's strategy about chores. But they still helped out around the house. Maria could feel the lessening of her caregiving role as she stopped doing everything for them and they learned to do things for themselves.

Nia's diagnosis changed that in many ways. There were so many things related to her cancer that Nia couldn't understand or do. In some ways, Maria felt like she was back to having a toddler again. Nia would struggle and cry, and Maria would comfort her. Nia was afraid and didn't understand everything that was happening. Maria had to find a way to explain things to Nia on her level and to support Nia in dealing with her fears.

As the treatments have become more of a routine, Maria is now watching Nia start to take back some of her independence. Maria is working to give Nia choices as much as possible. What does she want to do first? What does she want as a reward afterward? Maria's role as Nia's caregiver has changed, but as always she is doing her best to help her daughter.

Daniel in Intensive Care

After Daniel's second surgery, he spends several days in the pediatric intensive care unit (PICU). The hospital requests that a parent or guardian stay with Daniel 24/7 while he's in the PICU. Nana and Papa find this challenging since visitors are not allowed to eat in the PICU, and they are barely able to sleep given the frequent dinging and buzzing along with Daniel's anxiety outbursts.

Nana stays overnight with Daniel most nights. He often startles in bed, flailing his arms and crying out. For Nana, this is an entirely new type of caregiving. She wants to help, but she isn't sure what to do. She sits next to the bed and tries to soothe him. She sings to him, puts his favorite movies on the TV, and rubs his back. Neither of them gets much sleep over the course of three days in the PICU.

Once Daniel is discharged, it takes them both a while to sleep normally, even at home. Daniel continues to startle in the middle of the night and cry out for Nana. When Nana asks the doctor about it, he suggests that Daniel might suffer from post-intensive care syndrome. Nana ends up sleeping in Daniel's room for several weeks, darkening the shades, and doing her best to calm him before bed and when he wakes up. Daniel's needs had become much more intense, and his grandparents had to adjust their caregiving accordingly.

QUESTIONS TO ASK YOURSELF

- What are my child's current needs?
- How are those needs more, less, or different than a couple of years ago? How have my child's medical challenges changed their needs?
- How is my role as a caregiver right now different from what I thought it would be?
- How do I feel about being a caregiver at this stage of my child's life?

ACTION STEPS

- In your C.O.A.C.H. notebook, write down five words that describe how you feel about being a caregiver right now.
- Meet with a trusted person in your support network and chat about how you're feeling as a caregiver right now.

11

You Are the Leader of Your Child's Medical Team

> Great leaders are not the best at everything. They find people who are best at different things and get them all on the same team.
>
> —Eileen Bitrisky, leadership consultant

Reading the title of this chapter, you might be thinking, "What do you mean I have to be a leader? What does that have to do with medical trauma?"

Some of you were born to be leaders. But for others, the title of this chapter might make you want to run in the opposite direction. But wait! Wait! Stay with us. You already are a leader for your child. This chapter will help you understand why being the leader of your child's medical team is important, and it will give you some tools to help you manage this role.

Have you ever been in the hospital? If you have, then you've seen the mix of people who serve each patient. There are nurses, doctors, and therapists, and, more specifically, attending doctors, residents, charge nurses, night nurses, and so on. There are *a lot* of people involved in just one hospital stay.

Let's look at life outside the hospital for families of children with medical challenges. A child with a chronic condition could have ten or more different specialists that they see on a periodic basis.

Whether your child is in the hospital or just having regular doctor's appointments, there is no one who understands your child better than *you.*

"But wait," you might say. "My child's main doctor understands their condition much better than I do. They went to school for this, and they see hundreds of patients every year. I don't know as much as they do." This may be true. But your child is so much more than their medical condition.

You know how your child's medical challenges play out in your child's life every day at home. You know how they affect your child at school. You know which medications make your child tired or hyper and which ones give them a rash. You know that if a surgeon says it will take your child a week to recover, it will take longer. You know how they might respond to being stuck in the hospital or cooped up at home. You are the one who knows when they are feeling bad enough that you might need to call the doctor.

No one understands your child better than you.

Maybe you never looked at these situations as making you the leader. But your child looks to you for help, and your role is to lead the effort to help them.

So what does it look like to lead your child's medical team?

WHAT DO YOU WANT YOUR CHILD'S MEDICAL CARE TEAM TO LOOK LIKE?

Well, it's hard to put together a team and then lead it if you don't know where you're going. So let's start with creating a vision for your child's health care. Go back to chapter 3 and look at your child's medical journey and the possible paths it might take. Then, focus on the current stage of your child's journey and its possible future paths.

What are your child's goals at this stage of their life? Given any medical challenges, what will it take to reach them? What specific medical challenges are they facing? Do they need to heal from an injury? Do they need to learn to manage their own medications? Are you expecting additional surgeries? Are you working to have your child maintain their abilities as long as possible and have quality of life in the face of a terminal illness?

WHO SHOULD BE ON THE TEAM?

Once you have a general sense of the goals for your child, you can better identify who the medical and therapeutic team members might be. For most families, the team starts with their child's pediatrician. Depending on what your child needs, you might add specialists, therapists, and care facilities.

It might feel daunting to consider all the potential medical situations that might crop up. Try not to get caught up in the "what ifs." Start small. As you get used to leading your child's medical team, you'll be able to better consider different scenarios and be more prepared.

For now, look at your child's current providers. If your child has a specific medical condition, focus on that for a moment: Are there generally expected symptoms or complications for their condition? Does your child have all the providers they currently need? If you don't know, this is a great time to reach out to members of your support team or parents of children with similar conditions to identify providers who might be good choices for those situations.

Once you've put together *who* should be on your child's medical team, you might wonder, "What does it take to lead?"

HOW DOES LEADING MY CHILD'S MEDICAL TEAM AFFECT MEDICAL TRAUMA?

You may have noticed that we haven't talked very much about medical trauma in the last three chapters. You might have even asked yourself, "What does my identity have to do with helping my child through a surgery? Why does it matter how I view myself as a caregiver? Why do I need a vision for my child's health care?"

The answer is this: *you are the constant.* You are the lens through which your child will see many of their experiences, especially while they are young. You are the one who explains things to your child. Your child looks to you for cues as to whether something is good or bad, okay or not okay, funny or a waste of time.

You are the decision maker. You (and maybe a partner) will decide on the medical providers, the facilities, the medications, and the surgeries. You will have input on who comes in and out of your child's hospital room.

You are the leader of your child's medical team. Sometimes it might be necessary to ask questions or share your concerns with your child's medical team. Many parents experience reluctance or fear about these discussions. One research study reported that many parents of children with chronic medical conditions said that they only took charge after "medical professionals were unwilling or unable to meet the child's needs." This research also highlighted that parents are often afraid of being perceived negatively by health professionals if they express their opinions about their child's care in those scenarios.[1]

You are the constant. You are the decision maker. You are the leader of your child's medical team.

We're not going to sugarcoat it. Sometimes being a leader can create uncomfortable discussions with health care providers. Sometimes there is an imbalance of power that might cause a provider to get defensive if you step in and question their recommendation. Keep reading to learn about some tools to make this process easier.

Some parents choose to rely on their child's doctors' recommendations and decide not to ask questions but instead focus on coordinating their child's care. This is still a way to lead your child's team.

WHAT DOES LEADING MY CHILD'S MEDICAL TEAM LOOK LIKE?

Describing the challenges of parenting, Brené Brown states, "Like many of you, parenting is by far my boldest and most daring adventure."[2] This is certainly true when you are working to lead your child's medical care. Here are some ideas to keep in mind as you navigate this new terrain:

- **Knowledge:** Every team member has their area of expertise. Remember that you are the expert on your child. You bring knowledge about how medical situations and stress affect them.
- **Relationships:** Building a working relationship with your child's health care providers is important. Aim to be respectful and work with them to create the best plans and make the best decisions for your child's medical care. Tell them and show them when you appreciate something that they have done for your child.

- **Clarity:** Try to be clear with the team about the information you need, your child's needs, and the decisions you make.
- **Decisiveness:** If you are having a hard time making a decision about your child's care, ask your medical team for help. Involve your child in decisions if they are old enough and want to have a say.
- **Courage:** Parenting can be a tough gig. Some of the medical decisions that you make for your child might be hard. Sometimes you might feel that you need to ask questions or disagree with your medical team. Many parents find it takes courage to share these thoughts and opinions.
- **Passion:** Sometimes you might need your passion in caring for your child to carry you through. At times you might need to balance your passion with learning and patience.

Hopefully by now you realize that leading your child's medical team is just an extension of how you parent and care for them. Try not to let yourself feel intimidated! You are your child's best advocate and can share your unique expertise with the team.

Maria Speaks Up for Nia

Maria was very intimidated by Nia's oncologist (a doctor who specializes in treating cancer) when she first met him. He was a head taller than her and talked fast, but he was always kind and patient. When he first introduced the surgeon who would perform Nia's surgery to remove the tumor, Maria started to feel overwhelmed by the number of people involved. She would go on to meet the anesthesiologist and lots of nurses too. It seemed like a well-oiled machine, and Maria just nodded her head a lot of the time. And cried when she was alone.

After the surgery, it is time to start chemotherapy. Nia's oncologist tells Maria that the hospital will call with a schedule of all of Nia's upcoming appointments. When Maria receives the first phone call with a chemo schedule for Nia, she is not offered a choice of when to schedule appointments but instead is given a list of days and times and told not to be late. Maria looks over the list and starts to become overwhelmed, noting most of the appointments are scheduled for the early morning. As we learned earlier, Nia struggles when she feels rushed. Maria also knows she will have to change her work schedule to bring Nia to these appointments.

At first, Maria tries to make it work, resulting in stressful mornings. Nia grows more withdrawn and anxious as the treatments wear on. Maria finally gathers the courage to speak up to the doctor and is able to reschedule the treatments to a better time for Nia and her family (read more about timing in chapter 22). This is the first step that helps Maria gain confidence in voicing her perspective about treatment options and the logistics surrounding the appointments.

As their journey continues, Maria even looks into clinical trials that might be available. When Maria finds one that she thinks might help Nia, she talks to Nia's doctor, but this treatment isn't available at their hospital. Maria researches some more and reaches out to the contact for the clinical trial that she found. Nia's doctor also looks into it, and, together, they make a plan for the next steps of Nia's treatment.

New Decisions for Daniel

Daniel is now four years old. It's been almost a year since his diagnosis with Hunter syndrome. Recently, one of his doctors asked Nana and Papa if they had ever considered a stem cell transplant for Daniel's condition. This doctor is new to their local hospital. She had performed transplants on patients with conditions similar to Daniel's at her previous hospital.

This is a huge decision. On the one hand, the doctor seems confident that this option could really help Daniel, but it also comes with a significant risk of complications and even death. The other option is to continue with the treatments Daniel is already receiving and hope for even better ones down the road. No one can really tell Nana and Papa what to do since Daniel's condition is so rare and there isn't a lot of information about the best course of treatment.

Nana and Papa know they have to gather the information they need in order to best help Daniel. They speak to doctors about the process, which would involve a months-long stay in the hospital and being immunocompromised for an extended period. Daniel's anxiety over going to the hospital each week has started to subside, but they can't imagine being in the hospital for months and then keeping him away from people. They ask lots of questions of other parents who have been in similar situations.

Finally, they decide to continue with the treatment plan they had originally decided on with Daniel's main doctor. Given that the outcomes aren't certain and the risk is greater with the experimental therapy, they feel that sticking with the consistency and routine that they have already established with Daniel's treatment is the better option for him in the short term and hopefully the long term as well. They are grateful that Daniel's medical team supports their decision and continues to work to find ways to lessen Daniel's anxiety related to his hospital visits.

QUESTIONS TO ASK YOURSELF

- What are my child's goals?
- What are my goals for my child?
- Who is part of my child's medical team?
- During the past few medical situations I've had with my child, did it feel like I was on a team? Why or why not?

ACTION STEPS

- In your C.O.A.C.H. notebook, make a list of the members of your child's medical team.
- Consider your own knowledge, relationships, clarity, decisiveness, courage, and passion. Write down two strengths and two weaknesses you have in relation to these qualities. Consider how to grow in those weaker areas.

12

You Are a C.O.A.C.H.

> Coaches have to watch for what they don't want to see and listen to what they don't want to hear.
>
> —John Madden, former NFL football coach and sportscaster

We first introduced the C.O.A.C.H. process in chapter 3. Now that you've thought more about your identities as a person, a parent, a caregiver, and a leader of your child's medical team, we're going to get more specific about how that connects to your role as a C.O.A.C.H. for your child's medical trauma.

If you've ever played sports, you know that a coach can have a significant impact on their players. The coach can teach, encourage, motivate, and guide them. The coach observes them in order to figure out how to help. The coach helps them manage their disappointment.

The C.O.A.C.H. process builds those same principles into an easy-to-remember acronym. Here's a reminder of what it stands for:

Collect information.
Observe the situation.
Ask questions of yourself, your child, and professionals.
Choose the strategies.
Help your child, get help from others.

In earlier chapters, we've only touched on this process. Here, we'll go into more detail.

The C.O.A.C.H. process isn't always a linear process of step one, step two, step three, and so forth. Some of these steps will overlap, happen at the same time, and be repeated as you work to support your child. This acronym is designed to help you remember all the pieces that come together to help your child deal with medical trauma and health challenges.

Earlier in this book, we suggested creating a C.O.A.C.H. notebook, where you can include notes related to your child's medical care and potential medical trauma. You can create this either on paper or digitally. Having that one notebook you can grab off the shelf or access easily on your phone or tablet that compiles all these thoughts will be helpful over time.

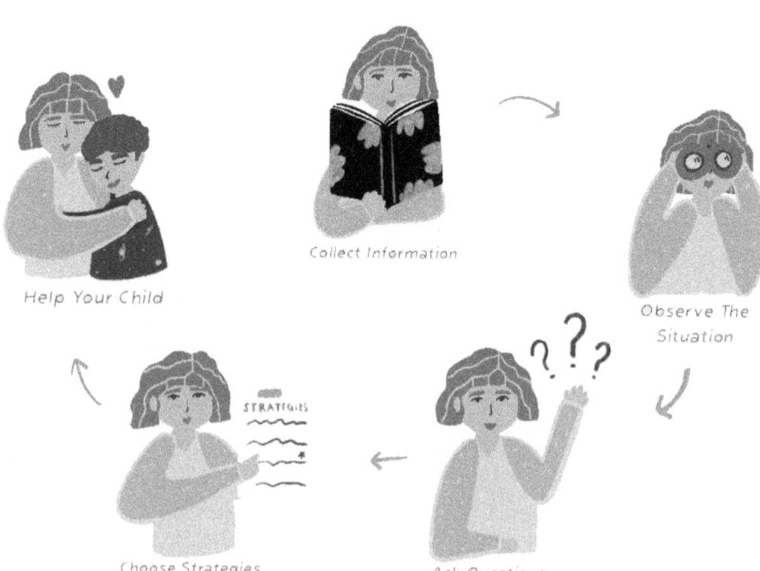

Figure 12.1. The C.O.A.C.H. Process

COLLECT INFORMATION

Medical situations can often feel overwhelming because of the sheer amount of new information being thrown at us. The terminology, the risks, and the unknowns can combine to jumble everything into a mess. So how do we take in this information in a way that is meaningful and helps us support our child?

Information gathering in medical situations often happens in three stages: before, during, and after medical events. If your child has an upcoming surgery or doctor's appointment, collect information beforehand in order to understand the who, what, where, when, why, and how:

- Who will be involved?
- What is expected to happen? Can someone explain it step by step?
- Where will it occur? What is the environment like?
- When will the procedure happen?
- Why do we need to do it?
- How is the procedure or appointment supposed to go?

Where can you find this information? Some of it will come from your child's medical providers. You might also have past experience with this provider, this location, or these types of procedures. You may be able to find additional reliable information online: look for trusted health care providers, institutions, and organizations that can offer additional information or ask your medical team for reputable websites. If your child has a chronic condition, disease organizations and/or other parents are also great sources of information about upcoming medical challenges.

Ask lots of questions. Ask yourself, ask your child, ask the medical providers.

Once you've collected information *before* a medical procedure, you and your child will be able to walk in with some level of preparedness. Once you're at the appointment, or at the hospital for surgery, you'll continue to collect information *during* that time. You'll learn more about what general practices are, who works well with your child, what makes your child nervous or comforts them, and how you yourself respond to these situations. Collecting information is an ongoing process.

When appointments or procedures are over, *after* the event, you will collect information that you learned. What worked? What didn't? Which providers are your child's favorites? What would you have changed?

Over time, you can figure out your own system for collecting information—the sources you trust, the questions you ask, and the important facts. You may want to keep this information in your notebook to make it easy to find.

OBSERVE THE SITUATION

Observing is one part of collecting information that we described above. There are several areas you may want to consider observing.

First, observe how your child responds to situations, people, pain, and environments. Noticing your child's responses will offer you key information about their potential for medical trauma and their actual experience of it. Watch them in their comfortable environment—at home, at school, at play. Observe how they respond in a medical environment. What changes about their demeanor (if anything)? Does how they talk or what they talk about change?

Second, observe the medical providers' interaction with your child. Who makes your child comfortable? How do they do that? What actions draw your child in or shut them down?

Third, observe the environment. Is it sterile or playful? White or colorful? Cold or warm (emotionally and physically)? What might it *feel* like to your child, and how does it differ from other environments they are used to?

ASK QUESTIONS

Ask lots of questions. Ask yourself, ask your child, ask the medical providers.

What should you ask yourself? What don't you know about the upcoming procedure? Is anything making you nervous? What can you do to find that information?

Asking your child questions is just as important. What do they know about the appointment? How do they feel about doctors?

About hospitals? Is there anything they'd like to know? Anything that would make it easier or more comfortable for them?

When it comes to asking questions of medical providers, sometimes parents feel intimidated. Or they don't want to waste the provider's time. Most medical providers are very open to questions. Most want you and your child to feel comfortable about their care. Before you head to a medical appointment, consider making a list of questions in your C.O.A.C.H. notebook.

Asking questions can be part of both collecting information and evaluating how best to help your child. That's why follow-up questions are important. For example, let's say that you ask the physician to describe a medical procedure to freeze a wart off of your child's finger. The doctor tells you that the freezing solution is cold and must be held on the wart for at least thirty seconds. Some great follow-up questions would be: Do most kids think it hurts? What has the doctor done in the past to distract children during that time? Will they have to do it more than once during a visit? Will it take more than one visit?

If you learn a little about the procedure before a medical appointment, it can help you identify some questions to ask. It can be helpful to ask your child's medical provider to confirm that they will perform the procedure in the way that you read about. Many providers do things differently. You can't necessarily count on appointments, tests, or procedures going exactly how they are described by a different provider or resource.

CHOOSE THE STRATEGIES

Especially as we consider preparing for a specific upcoming medical appointment, the steps of collecting information, observing the situation, and asking questions can be used together to better understand the medical challenge your child is facing. Knowing what to expect can help you choose which strategies you will use to support your child.

We'll describe a number of different strategies in the next section of the book. You might find that you want to use several of them regularly. Others may be particularly helpful in supporting specific medical challenges. Keep in mind that you don't have to do everything.

You can select the one or two strategies that you think will work best for each situation.

Focusing on one or two particular strategies will also help you learn how these make the experience (hopefully) better for your child. You may be able to include additional strategies for the next medical challenge. You will also find out which strategies don't seem to work for your child, in which case you will know to try something different next time.

As you learn about each strategy in the next section of the book, consider taking notes in your C.O.A.C.H. notebook. This might help you consider all your options for each upcoming medical visit.

HELP YOUR CHILD

The ultimate goal of the C.O.A.C.H. process is to help your child. Once you've collected information, observed your child and the situation, asked questions, and selected strategies to try, you can take steps to help your child. Some strategies involve a process, some involve changing current household or parenting practices, and some are specific experiences with your child.

It may not be obvious right away if a strategy is making a difference to prevent or reduce medical trauma. Consider making notes about your child's reactions and experiences in your C.O.A.C.H. notebook so that you can look at what happens over time. And sometimes, as they say, no news is good news. If your child *isn't* acting out or throwing tantrums about medical procedures, and they seem to deal with their medical care more like daily life, this is a *good thing*.

So now that you've become more familiar with the C.O.A.C.H. process, let's see it in action with two of our families.

C.O.A.C.H.ing Nia

When Nia first starts chemo, her appointments are at 8:00 a.m. on Tuesdays and last several hours. Maria arranges to take Tuesday mornings off from work. Nia's grandmother stays with her at home on Tuesday afternoons. A few weeks into chemo, on a Saturday morning, Nia starts complaining about her stomach. She starts withdrawing more, not wanting to talk with her friends or hang out with her family. That Monday, Nia begs her mother to stay home from school. On her way to chemo the next day, she doesn't want to eat before the visit, and she doesn't talk much. Maria knows that Nia is going through a lot but is not sure what is causing Nia's emotional changes.

Maria remembers that she can use the C.O.A.C.H. process to try to support Nia. Maria starts *collecting* information by reading and asking the doctor more questions about the medication Nia is receiving and how it might make her feel. She also calls Nia's teacher and asks about how Nia is doing at school. She learns that Nia is often anxious and that when people ask why she has to miss school, she doesn't respond.

Maria *observes* how Nia responds at the next appointment. Maria sees Nia wince when they stick her for the IV. Nia wants the curtains closed and doesn't eat even though Maria brought her favorite snacks. While Nia says her stomach is fine, Maria now knows that the medication can make her stomach upset.

Maria starts *asking* more questions. She asks if the nurse has anything available to help numb Nia's skin before inserting the IV. She asks Nia if it upsets her when kids ask her about missing school. She asks Nia if she wants to cook or play together before her appointments to keep her mind occupied.

Maria *chooses* a few strategies to help Nia manage her medical trauma. She changes the timing of her appointments (read more in chapter 22). She communicates better with Nia (read more in chapter 15). She offers cooking and playing as a distraction (read more in chapter 23). She also adapts the environment by bringing some fun posters to hang on the curtain in their space at the hospital (read more in chapter 21).

Together, all of these strategies *help* Nia make her hospital days more of what she wants, less painful, and more tolerable.

C.O.A.C.H.ing Daniel

Nana and Papa have gotten into a good routine with Daniel's weekly hospital visits for infusions and the routine doctor visits every six months or so. But in about a month, Daniel is scheduled for surgery on his hands. They are concerned since he had a really difficult time with the anesthesia mask before his last surgery. He also pulled at the tubes and IV line afterward. Even after he'd left the pediatric intensive care unit and come home, recovery was rough.

Daniel's grandparents are determined to make this stay a better one by learning what they can and by planning ahead. They start by *collecting* information about the surgery and expected recovery process, including alternatives for anesthesia.

They remember *observing* Daniel not liking being surprised that a mask was coming toward his face and not expecting the tubes and other lines.

They *ask* the medical team about how anesthesia could be done differently, explaining Daniel's trauma from the previous surgery. They also ask about how to hide the tubes and make them less accessible to Daniel. Finally, they ask specific questions about the casts he will have to wear after the surgery, whether the doctor had any that they could use in medical play, and how they can make them less scary and more fun for him (by using colored casts, decorating them, etc.).

They *choose* to plan ahead, create a teaching story about the surgery (see more about this in chapter 18), and to use medical play (see chapter 20) for Daniel to have an opportunity to play out his anticipated anesthesia and then recovery from the surgery.

By the time surgery day comes, Daniel is talking about the mask and how he is going to hold it on his face and how he can't wait to wear his superhero gloves after the hospital. Nana and Papa are so excited that it seems like the strategies they chose may really *help* prevent more trauma to Daniel from the surgery.

QUESTIONS TO ASK YOURSELF

- How have I collected information about my child's care in the past? Am I using reliable sources?
- What have I already learned about my child's medical care by observing my child, their health care providers, and the medical environment?
- Do I regularly ask questions of my child's medical providers, or do I just listen to what they have to say?

ACTION STEPS

- In your C.O.A.C.H. notebook, create a section to write down information and notes related to your child's medical care and medical trauma strategies.
- Consider your child's most recent medical event and walk through the C.O.A.C.H. process as if it were happening now. Consider writing out the C.O.A.C.H. process as it applies to your child.

Part 4

STRATEGIES FOR PREVENTING AND REDUCING MEDICAL TRAUMA

13

General Strategies

Parenting Children with Medical Conditions

Trust yourself. You know more than you think you do.

—Dr. Benjamin Spock

Thinking about how to support your child through their medical journey (while also on your own journey) may be overwhelming at times. For many parents, thoughts pile up and swirl around when they discover a new medical condition in their child or when they learn about a change in a medical condition. Sometimes even the "simple" task of taking your child for routine medical care can keep you up at night worrying.

We provide some specific strategies in this book to help guide parents in supporting their child and themselves; these strategies are intended to build on what you already do as a parent.

In chapter 2, we introduced some common parenting styles: authoritarian, authoritative, permissive, and uninvolved. What is your typical parenting style? Knowing this will help you as you figure out how to support your child on their medical journey. Think about how you handle any challenges with your child. When you are faced with a new medical challenge, you can first try parenting strategies that you know have worked for your child in other situations. For example, if your child is afraid, do you provide them with information? Give them hugs? Bring them a favorite toy? Distract them? One of these strategies may work to help your child through a medical challenge that they are afraid of.

Here are a few other general strategies that may be helpful:

1. **Break it down into smaller pieces.** A new medical condition can be very overwhelming. To start helping your child in their medical journey, it may help to break the big picture down into smaller parts, both for your child and yourself. For example, once you learn of your child's diagnosis, you can slowly provide your child with information, depending on their age and personality. For young children, naming their medical condition and telling them what to expect that day or the next may be enough. Some older children want all the information, while others just want the basics. Some children prefer to learn about their diagnosis in small pieces. As a parent, you also may have many questions and decisions to make. Write down everything that comes to your mind, then divide it up into categories:
    - Needs attention immediately
    - Needs attention within the next day or so
    - Needs attention this week
    - Handle this later
2. **Be there for your child.** It sounds simple, but being there for your child is one of the most powerful tools you have. Spend time with your child. Put your phone, computer, tablet, or book down. Be there for the stuff that is most difficult for your child. That doesn't mean that you must be there every minute of every day. Instead, be sure your child knows that they can count on you when they need you. If you need some time to yourself (which we highly recommend) or need to go to work, make sure that your child has someone they can call if they need help. Depending on your child's age, this could be you via phone, or family, friends, or someone on the medical team, such as a nurse.

    There is no one-size-fits-all approach to parenting a child through a medical condition.

3. **Be honest with your child.** If you are facing a long medical journey, one of the most important things you can do is ensure your child can trust you. Being honest about their medical condition helps to build this trust. Decide what your child needs

to know about their medical condition. This will be different depending on your child's age, cognitive abilities, and personality. We recommend that you share the name of your child's medical condition (otherwise they will overhear it) and how it will directly affect them. Your medical team can help you with this if you aren't sure what to share or how to talk to your child about their condition.

4. **Make decisions based on your child and your family.** There is no one-size-fits-all approach to parenting a child through a medical condition. You are likely to have many people tell you exactly what you "should" do in your situation. Take the advice that is helpful and leave the rest. For example, when you are deciding how much information to share, some children like to know as much detail as possible, while others prefer for their parents to handle it all and just tell them exactly what will affect them in the moment. What feels normal in your family? If you have a vacation coming up, do you tell your child everything about it so they can prepare? Or do you tell them the plan day by day or hour by hour? Consider also how you process information: Are you an information seeker? Do you prefer to deal with things one step at a time? Use both your own and your child's preferences in deciding how much to share with your child and when to share it.
5. **Give yourself time.** New medical challenges are exactly that: challenges. As with any new adventure or twist and turn in life, these challenges will take time to adjust to. Many parents have shared that when they first learned of a new diagnosis, they shut down and don't remember anything else from that conversation. This is normal. Take the time you need; learn slowly over time.
6. **Do your best and let go of the rest.** Hindsight is twenty-twenty. Looking back, you can always think of something you could have done a little bit better. Try to look forward, do your best, love your child, and let go.

Sharing with Cameron

In the immediate weeks to months following the accident, Cameron's parents were overwhelmed, exhausted, and hoping things would just go back to normal. However, his recovery has been more intense physically and emotionally than his family and he had expected. His emotional reactions were a particular surprise as he had never had challenges with his emotions in the past.

At first, Cameron's parents tried to protect him by limiting the amount of information that they shared with Cameron. For example, when they learned that he had to have another surgery, they didn't tell him until the night before. However, keeping information from Cameron actually increased his anxiety—he knows his parents well and sensed they were hiding something from him. His mind created all kinds of reasons why they wouldn't tell him what was going on. He became afraid that he was going to lose his legs and thought maybe that was why they were being secretive.

One evening, Cameron breaks down and starts crying and tells his mother, Zoe, his fears. Zoe realizes that it would be better to share more of his recovery information with him as they learn it. As a family, they are typically very open about challenges and work together to deal with tough things. Cameron's parents realize that they should take this same approach in helping him deal with his medical condition.

Another challenge that Cameron is facing is related to his medical trauma avoidance symptoms. This contributes to him not listening to his parents and not getting ready for school in a timely fashion. His parents tend to parent differently from one another with his mother tending toward a more authoritative style and his father generally being more permissive. When his father tries to let Cameron lead the way in getting ready for school (like he did before the accident), everyone ends up yelling and being late to start their day.

In this instance, Cameron's parents decide that they need to take a more authoritative approach. In the past, Zoe had created chore checklists with rewards to help motivate Cameron. Zoe and Preston decide to start a reward system (discussed more in chapter 17) for Cameron getting ready for school on time. While this doesn't solve the problem entirely due to his ongoing medical trauma, it does help Cameron begin to get back on track with getting ready in the morning.

Sharing with Nia and Sara

When Nia's mother, Maria, first learned that Nia had cancer, she was devastated. She didn't know what to tell Nia or her sister. Maria's friends and family gave her all kinds of advice. Some friends told her not to use the word *cancer* around Nia or her sister, Sara, because it might scare them. Other friends told her that she needed to share everything with Nia right away so she would know what to expect.

Maria thought about both of her children carefully in deciding what to share. She knew that Nia would probably become very overwhelmed with too much information. Nia likes to know what is going on in the moment; she has a hard time keeping things straight if she's given too much information at once. However, Sara always wants to know exactly what is going on and what the plan is. She does better when she knows what to expect. Maria asks the medical team for help explaining just the basics of Nia's cancer to her. She also asks that they talk outside the room so that she can choose to share small pieces of information with Nia over time. Maria also wants to be sure that Sara can ask any questions she has away from her sister, so she finds a separate time to talk with Sara. Because Maria is often with Nia at appointments or the hospital, she gives Sara a notebook where she can write down questions as she thinks of them.

Maria makes her own plan for her family. She listens to advice from others, but she does what she thinks is best in the end.

QUESTIONS TO ASK YOURSELF

- What types of parenting strategies work best with my child?
- How do I handle conflicting parenting advice?
- What level of information does my child prefer to know about topics such as medical care or their condition?

ACTION STEPS

- In your C.O.A.C.H. notebook, write down a recent parenting success story.
- Is there something overwhelming about your child's medical condition? Write it down and try breaking it into steps.

14

Planning Ahead

Planning Makes . . . Better

It takes as much energy to wish as it does to plan.

—Eleanor Roosevelt

We all know that the old saying "planning makes perfect" isn't true, especially when children are involved. But some planning can definitely help to reduce stress for both children and parents. Most children do better when they have an idea about what to expect. They may not need to know every detail (though some children request this), but having a general sense of what their day and/or week will look like can be helpful. In planning, think about (1) timing, (2) stuff, and (3) communication.

TIMING

While medical appointments, procedures, and hospitalizations are usually disruptive to a child's and family's typical day, you can minimize disruption and distress when you take your child's preferences and needs into account. When you are scheduling or preparing for medical appointments or procedures, take a minute to consider your child's typical schedule and routines. Here are some questions for you to think about:

- What time does your child usually wake up?
- Is your child an early riser, or is getting them up in the morning like trying to wake a bear from hibernation?
- Does your child take a rest or a nap in the afternoon?
- Is your child an energizer bunny with a need to run around?
- Are there holidays, school events, or other activities that are particularly important to your family?
- What are your child's eating routines?
- How does eating—or not eating—affect your child's behaviors?
- What does your child like to eat?

If you ask a group of parents about the most common reasons for cranky kids, two things are bound to come up: my child is tired, and my child is hungry. Sometimes it is inevitable that your child will be hungry or tired at a medical appointment. Other times, planning ahead may be able to prevent this.

If there is flexibility in scheduling and you know your child hates getting up early in the morning, consider scheduling an appointment later in the day. Similarly, if your child naps, try to avoid naptime appointments. No one wants tired kids at appointments when it can be helped (this includes your child's nurses and doctors!).

In planning, think about (1) timing, (2) stuff, and (3) communication.

If your child is in the hospital and requires morning treatments but prefers to sleep later in the morning (this is very commonly the case with teenagers), ask to schedule treatments as late as possible. Similarly, medical teams often do rounds early in the morning; if they do not need to directly examine your child at that time, ask to step out in the hall for morning rounds to allow your child to sleep.

When you think of the timing of appointments, you may also want to consider your child's energy level. If you have a child who has a need to move, you will want to either (a) minimize the amount of time they are in the waiting room (get the earliest appointment possible) or (b) schedule appointments so that you have time before for your child to jump their energy out at home first. You may also want to find out approximately how long you will need to entertain your child in an exam room, how long patients often have to wait, and/or how long your child will be in the hospital ahead of time. Before you go, try to learn about playrooms or areas to walk to if you have time.

Then there is the food factor. Bring plenty of foods and snacks with you. Assume the appointment or procedure will take twice as long as you expect, and bring enough food for your child and yourself. If you have a kid who is cranky when they haven't eaten and they aren't allowed to eat before an appointment or procedure, request the earliest possible appointment time and pack food to give them as soon as it is allowed. Try to avoid eating in front of your child or cooking strong-smelling foods before the appointment. But don't forget to feed yourself. Trying to navigate a medical appointment as a cranky parent with a hungry kid is rough.

Some appointments and procedures are time sensitive and must happen right away, but others may be flexible. For those that aren't emergencies, look at your calendar and see if there are holidays or events that you want to try to avoid. For example, if your child's birthday is coming up, would it be better to do a procedure before or after? If you plan to have a party, how can you coordinate that with the required medical care? Or if your child wants to attend a particular sports event or school play, is there a way to make it work with their medical care? If you are unsure about how quickly a procedure or an appointment needs to happen, ask your child's medical team.

In the midst of considering the timing of medical events for your child, it is also important to consider your own needs. For example, if there is flexibility in scheduling, are there certain days of the week or times of day that are less stressful for you? Parents may need to consider work schedules, schedules of other children, traffic patterns, and transportation needs when planning for appointments. See chapter 22 for more tips on timing.

THE STUFF

The stuff. Oh so much stuff when you are going anywhere with kids! A medical appointment or a trip to the hospital can be like a trip to the zoo, only not quite as fun. It can be colder or warmer than expected, take way longer than you thought it would, and take unexpected turns. By packing what you may need, the trip can go much more smoothly and be less stressful, no matter what happens at the appointment. A packing list may include any of the following:

- favorite toys
- games
- art supplies
- a favorite stuffed animal or doll
- a favorite blanket
- electronic devices (e.g., tablets, phones, and their associated charging cords)
- extra clothes
- food
- medications
- special medical supplies

COMMUNICATION

Let your child know what to expect. Imagine that you get up one day with a plan to go to work, but then your best friend shows up and says that instead you are going to the hospital for a surgery. That probably wouldn't go over very well for you. Similarly, it is not helpful to throw something that could be stressful on your child at the last minute. How much in advance you tell your child and how much information to give them will depend on your child's age and needs. It can be helpful to share your plan. You may even be able to include your child in the plan. You can ask your child to help pack or choose toys and snacks for the day. See chapter 15 for more tips on communication.

Jin Goes to the Pediatrician

As we've learned, even routine medical appointments can be a challenge for Jin. Jin's parents are already dreading her five-year-old well-check appointment, which is scheduled for a month from now. Since Jin started working with a speech therapist and a pediatric psychologist, things have been going better. She is more comfortable with her daily diabetes monitoring and treatment. She's also done pretty well at her medical appointments. But her parents know Jin needs her flu shot at this appointment and that she will remember this office from the last shots she had. Amy and Cole hope that some of the work they've done with Jin related to her insulin shots will make these appointments better too, but they are unsure.

When Amy calls to schedule the well-check, she asks for the first appointment in the morning. Jin is an early riser, rarely sleeping later than six o'clock. She thinks that Jin will do better if she can get the appointment out of the way so she won't have to worry about it the whole day. Because Jin tends to worry a lot about her medical appointments and often becomes upset even thinking about shots, her parents wait to tell her until the day before the appointment. When they tell her, Jin starts yelling that she doesn't want to go and runs to her room, slamming the door. Her parents let her settle for a few moments and then ask Jin to help pack a special bag to take to the appointment. Together, they plan that Jin will get extra electronic time while she waits for the appointment and on the way home from the appointment. Jin picks out the shows she wants to watch on her tablet. Jin also chooses to take her favorite stuffed dog with her.

The morning of the appointment, Jin's parents try to keep her routine as normal as possible. They make sure that Jin eats ahead of time, and they pack a snack in case the doctor is running late. Jin still says that she doesn't want to go and cries as she gets in the car, but with her mom getting her show ready to watch, she does get in the car (which is an improvement). Jin still cries and screams right before the shot, but she is able to make it through the rest of the appointment better than before. After the appointment, Jin tells her parents that it wasn't that bad, despite the fact she had screamed through it. Jin's parents still feel worn out afterward, but they are encouraged that this appointment was a little better than the last.

Daniel's Hospitalization

We learned a little about Daniel's upcoming hand surgery in chapter 12 and how his grandparents tried to learn as much as possible about the surgery and the hospital stay in order to make it easier on Daniel. They also knew they had to plan ahead many of the logistics in order for the appointment to go smoothly.

At first, the hospital tells them that the surgery will be at 1:00 p.m. Knowing that Daniel won't be able to eat or drink all morning before his surgery, Nana makes a few calls and reschedules the surgery to 9:00 a.m. on a different day. She feels like they can keep Daniel busy and distracted from eating until they leave for the hospital at 7:00 a.m. but not all morning.

The day before, Nana packs all the things they'll need for the hospital—snacks for them and Daniel, his tablet, his favorite stuffed animal (a giraffe named Lolly), his photo book of friends, diapers and wipes since Daniel is not toilet trained, a change of clothes, the forehead thermometer and pulse oximeter that Daniel is used to at home, and even a separate backpack of overnight items in case something happens and they need to spend the night. Nana sets the coffeemaker for the morning and hides food and drinks that are normally on the counter so Daniel won't see them in the morning and feel even more hungry or thirsty.

Papa also sits down with Daniel to remind him they are going to the hospital the next day. He reads Daniel a teaching story (see chapter 18) that he had been reading to him each night for the past week to explain the soft casts Daniel will have on his hands after the surgery. Papa also tells Daniel that after the hospital, they will go get ice cream.

When Daniel finally goes to bed, Nana and Papa feel prepared for the surgery tomorrow.

QUESTIONS TO ASK YOURSELF

- When have my child's medical appointments or procedures gone the most smoothly? When have they gone the worst?
- What parts of my child's medical plan are within my control?

ACTION STEPS

- Look at your calendar for upcoming medical appointments. Decide if there are any appointments that you can and want to change.
- In your C.O.A.C.H. notebook, create your own personal packing list for your child's next doctor's appointment or hospital visit.

15

Communication

Let's Talk about It

The single biggest problem in communication is the illusion it has taken place.

—George Bernard Shaw

One common and frustrating experience of parents of children with medical challenges relates to communication,[1] yet communicating effectively about your child's medical condition is incredibly important.[2] Communicating information within the family, between the family and the medical team, and within the medical team is vital, but sometimes it's an epic disaster.

COMMUNICATION WITH THE MEDICAL TEAM

Trying to communicate with your child's medical team can be a journey in itself. This can be particularly challenging if your child's medical condition requires multiple specialties and/or hospitalizations.

There are a few strategies you can use to help ease communication challenges with the medical team:

1. **Ask questions.** You are your child's best advocate. You know your child better than any medical provider. If you aren't sure

about something, ask. If you aren't sure about the answer, ask again or ask a trusted team member. Some parents might worry about "bothering the doctors" or that the medical team might think they are that *difficult* parent. We encourage you to try to let go of those concerns if you have them. Many providers don't mind answering questions, and, in fact, part of their job is to help you understand what they are doing to care for your child.

2. **Try to identify a point of contact** (a person on the child's medical team) who can help coordinate your child's care and who you can regularly talk to about questions or updates about your child's care. This can be a go-to person for when you need information or don't understand something about your child's care.
3. **Ask for important information in writing.** This can help to ensure that the medical team has given you all the information that they intended to provide, to help you remember all the important stuff, and to help you share the information with other medical team members.

If your child is in the hospital, you are often meeting many different and changing medical teams. Even the very best doctors sometimes take a different approach to medical care. This can be particularly challenging when your child is in the hospital and needs multiple specialists or their doctor changes with every shift or every week. Here are some communication tips for when your child is in the hospital:

1. **Get visual.** Use the whiteboard or posterboard taped to the wall to post your questions and write down the responses you get while the doctor is in the room. This can help ensure you get your questions answered. It can show the doctors if there is a miscommunication and show other doctors what you have been told.
2. **Show your nurses some love.** Get to know each of your child's nurses and treat them well. In addition to the care nurses provide for your child, they are often key advocates for your child and can help you get answers to questions.
3. **Post your contact info.** If you need to leave your child's hospital room, post a *large note* with your phone number and "Please

call with updates and any changes to the medical plan." Ask your child's nurse to have the doctor call you every time they evaluate your child. Many parents need to work, help with siblings, or take a break when their child is in the hospital, and they're afraid to miss important information while they're away. This can help.

COMMUNICATION IN THE FAMILY

Sometimes it can be tough to maintain communication among family members (e.g., spouses, multiple caregivers, grandparents, siblings). Introducing a medical challenge into a family adds significant stress, including managing emotional reactions and often new logistical challenges. At a time when a family often needs to communicate *more* to keep things together, the added stress and responsibilities can sometimes have the opposite effect. Following are some ideas to combat this challenge:

1. **Hold weekly meetings.** Schedule a weekly family meeting with anyone who needs to be there. This can include your child, siblings, grandparents, parents, and/or others who are helping out a lot (e.g., neighbors, friends, aunts or uncles). This meeting could take place in person, via phone or video chat, or even through group text messaging if necessary. If it feels too much for you to manage, ask someone else to coordinate or run this meeting for your family. Run through the things that you need help with for the week and check in on how everyone is doing. You may also consider a small family meeting with just caregivers or just your child and their siblings.
2. **Write it down, and pass it around.** Unlike in school, where you might get in trouble for note passing, writing notes can be a big help here. Use a binder or journal that goes with your child to all medical appointments. Ask for printed summaries from each appointment or for a medical team member to check what you've written down to make sure your instructions are correct prior to leaving the appointment. Keep this binder with your child so that whoever is caring for them has the most up-to-date information.

Marriages and partnered relationships can take a hit during a child's medical challenge. Often one partner is tasked with much of the caregiving while the other is juggling many other life responsibilities. Ensure that you carve out time to connect with one another (easier said than done!). Consider a regular date night or a daily fifteen-minute check-in. Try to include time in which you talk about things other than your child with special medical needs or your other children.

COMMUNICATION WITH YOUR CHILD

The medical world can seem very scary to a child. There are lots of adults talking and moving and often using big words. The instruments they use may be things a child has never seen before with names they can't pronounce (and in reality, we may have never heard of them either). It can be difficult to talk with your child about medical challenges and to support them if you are practically speaking different languages—adult versus child.

It is important to establish a common language with your child surrounding medical care. What do they call these supplies? The medical instruments? What do they call various procedures or interactions?

To help your child communicate about their medical care, identify the terms that they use for medical people, places, and things. If you use visual supports with your child, name the items or activities featured on them with simple language (read more about visual supports in chapter 18). Using the words that your child uses can help you and your child discuss interventions that happened or will happen. It helps your child label and communicate about what hurt or made them anxious. Settling on common language around medical care with your child will be invaluable.

The medical world can seem very scary to a child.

The best language is descriptive and short, ideally one to three words at most. Longer descriptions will be harder for children, especially young or cognitively impaired children, to remember and use. For example, an infusion could be called "treatment," a stethoscope could be called a "scope," a needle could be called a "poke," and so on.

Once you and your child settle on some common terms, communicating about these topics will become easier.

Cameron and His Family Open Up

From what we know about Cameron so far, it is no surprise that his family struggled with communication right after his injury and during his early recovery. Cameron and his father, Preston, had similar reactions following the car accident and his injury: they both withdrew and communicated less. Cameron's mother, Zoe, was left to try to manage most of Cameron's medical care and recovery while also trying to make sure things didn't fall apart at home and at work.

Part of Cameron's communication challenges were directly related to medical trauma: he didn't want to talk about anything that reminded him of the accident and was having fears related to being in a car. Rather than communicating about his fears, he tried to avoid the car, which created all kinds of challenges in his family, as we described in chapter 13.

Now, three months after the accident, Zoe is at a loss as to how to support Cameron emotionally because he refuses to talk about the accident or about anything else that is bothering him. She believes he is having medical trauma reactions, and she takes him for therapy to help him learn skills to deal with his fears. She also asks the therapist to advise her on how to better support him.

Cameron is furious at first and does not want to go to therapy; however, after the first few sessions, he realizes (to his surprise) that it is actually starting to help him. Though he still doesn't want to talk about things much—he had never liked to talk much about feelings—he is learning ways to signal to his parents that he is having a tough time, and they are finding ways to support him.

At the same time, Preston and Zoe are struggling with a bit of a rough patch. Cameron's injuries and recovery are taking a toll on everyone. Everyone's stress level is high, and Zoe feels that Preston is not emotionally supporting the family. Preston is frustrated because he feels that his dedication to work and financial support of the family should be enough.

After a yelling match one evening, they both recognize how challenging the recent months have been in dealing with their initial fears that Cameron wouldn't survive the accident. The challenges with his recovery and the guilt they have both felt in not keeping him safe are also having an impact. They realize that in order to work together, they need to try to carve out time to talk with one another about how to manage this unique stage of their lives and family. They start with fifteen minutes on the phone a few times each week during their lunch breaks, talking about managing household tasks and activities. Over time (this takes several months, and there are a number of bumps in the road), Zoe and Preston are able to reconnect with one another to work better as a team and to better support each other.

Communicating during Nia's Hospital Stay

Throughout Nia's treatment, her family struggles to communicate with the medical team. Nia's mother, Maria, is often overwhelmed with the complexities of her medical care but is afraid to share this with the medical team. She finds staying in touch with Nia's doctors when Nia is in the hospital particularly tough because Maria has to work to keep Nia's medical insurance and to pay bills at home. She also has to care for Nia's sister, Sara.

Maria has asked the medical team to call her when they check on Nia, but they do not always remember. The medical team comes at a different time every day, so Maria never knows when she can ask questions.

Maria hates leaving Nia alone during the day at the hospital and is worried that the nurses think she is a bad mother. She is afraid to question the doctors even when she can tell Nia is behaving differently or seems to be in pain.

Fortunately for Nia and Maria, one of the oncologists taking care of Nia spends some time with her one afternoon, learning about the challenges that Maria is having juggling all her responsibilities to care for her children. This doctor comes to better understand Maria's situation and works with Maria to help improve communication. This doctor encourages Maria to ask questions at any time and suggests that she post her cell phone number in the hospital room so that any medical team member can call her if necessary.

Maria starts asking the doctor to write everything down. This helps her remember everything that she needs to do when they leave the hospital, and it is especially helpful when new doctors arrive for the next shift. Because Maria can be nervous around new medical team members, she finds it easier to show them what the doctor wrote down rather than explain everything verbally. While there are still times when communication between the medical team and Nia's family isn't perfect, Maria learns that she has the power to help with this communication and that it helps both Nia and the medical team with Nia's care.

QUESTIONS TO ASK YOURSELF

- Is my child's medical care more stressful because of communication challenges?
- Who are the people that I most need to communicate important information about my child's medical care with?
- What are the ways that I currently communicate about my child (or other important things) that seem to work well?
- What are some terms that my child uses to describe medical supplies, procedures, or devices?

ACTION STEPS

- Identify a trusted medical team member who can be your go-to for questions or concerns about your child's medical care.
- In your C.O.A.C.H. notebook, make a list of the common medical personnel, supplies, devices, and appointments/procedures and the terminology your child already uses. Consider any additional common language your child needs for these items.
- Choose a communication strategy from this chapter (or create a new one yourself!) to try for the next month.

16

Consistency

Knowing What to Expect

Expect the unexpected.

—Unknown

In general, kids (and often adults) do better when they know what to expect. Even in infants, consistent responses can help their development.[1] When we know what to expect, we can start making a plan about what to do, even if we don't like it. Knowing what to expect helps to take away the "what ifs."

Not knowing what to expect and constantly asking "what if?" can be some of the most difficult challenges when a child has a medical condition. Whether the medical condition is new or has been there for many years, the unknowns on your family's journey can be tough to navigate. For those with a new diagnosis, there may be a sudden change in life, shifting the way everything was done before. For those with a chronic condition, additional adjustments may be required every time something doesn't go as originally planned.

Parents may be tasked with trying to create consistency within unpredictability. This is no easy task. When things start to become overwhelming or seem to be changing constantly, it can be helpful to think about what you can and can't control. The things that we can't control are things to try to let go of (easier said than done, we know) or to put aside for the moment. This allows us more space to work on what we *can* control.

Think about the routines your family follows when things are going well—either before your child's medical challenge or at a time when your child's medical treatment was going well. There may be elements from these routines that you can bring into your child's current medical care.

Consistency doesn't have to be perfect. You can work with what you have in front of you. Maybe you always bring the same special snack, favorite stuffed animal, or favorite game to medical appointments. Maybe you keep the same bedtime routine at the hospital that you have at home. Or you video call your child from their hospital room into a family dinner at home. Maybe your child listens to the same music during every medical procedure or gets a treat once a procedure is complete.

Work on what you can control.

If you have other people in your child's life who help support them (e.g., coparent, spouse, grandparent, other family members), try to get everyone to use the same strategies to support your child through medical appointments and procedures. Even if the medical care is not predictable, how you help your child can be.

Adapting Daniel's Routines for Medical Care

Daniel was only three years old when his family learned of his Hunter syndrome diagnosis, but he had been seeing doctors for some time before that. He had even had one surgery. So Daniel's grandparents have been part of managing the ups and downs of his journey for years. We also learned earlier that Daniel began having more struggles with medical trauma and his behaviors after several months of infusions. Earlier in this book, we discussed a number of strategies that his grandparents used to help him with his medical trauma symptoms, including a picture schedule, medical play, and reward charts.

Daniel has now become very sensitive to changes in his schedule, and his medical care is only partially predictable. Sometimes he is sick and his medical team has to delay infusions. Sometimes the length of time that the infusions take varies based on reactions to his medication. While both grandparents try to attend every appointment, there are times when one of them has to take care of other family responsibilities or their own needs. Daniel also has a favorite nurse, and his anxiety substantially increases when she isn't there.

While many of the obstacles that Daniel is facing in the context of his medical treatment are not things that his grandparents can control, they take care to create consistency around his care wherever possible. For example, Daniel has a specific bedtime routine at home, which includes watching his favorite show, brushing his teeth, reading a book, and snuggling with his favorite stuffed animal, Lolly. When he has to stay overnight at the hospital, Daniel's grandparents follow the same routine as much as possible. They bring a tablet with his favorite shows downloaded, pack his favorite toothbrush, pick out books to pack for overnights, and bring Lolly. They try to keep the same bedtime regardless of whether he is at home or at the hospital.

Daniel's grandparents also work hard to develop a consistent routine for his infusions. On the way to the hospital, they play his favorite music. In the waiting room, he gets to choose a game on his tablet. During his port access, Nana holds his tablet up where he can watch it to help distract him. During the infusion, they work on art projects and play games together.

Even though his family cannot control Daniel's treatment or disease progression, they find that the routines they have put in place are comforting to Daniel.

New Routines for Cameron's Family

Cameron's injury was a totally unexpected, sudden change that affected his entire family. Prior to his injury, Cameron's life and his family's life were fairly uneventful. Cameron went to school, earned good grades, had friends, played on the soccer team, and only fought with his brother occasionally. His brother and parents also were doing well. His younger brother was following in his footsteps, both academically and on the soccer field. His parents both worked and got along well. They all had their routines: school/work, kids' sport practices and games, homework, and family dinners. On the weekend, Cameron spent a lot of time with friends and family.

After Cameron's injury, he was unable to quickly return to his routines. His hospitalization was longer than expected, as he had multiple complications from his surgeries. Rehab was taking months, and Cameron's emotional reactions were getting in the way of returning to the life and relationships he had before the accident.

He was devastated to learn that he might not be able to regain his pre-accident soccer skills.

Cameron's parents approached this differently, with his father catering to his needs, possibly out of guilt, and his mother pushing him to stay on track with his therapies in order to heal and recover. Zoe found herself arguing with Cameron daily over completing his exercises and homework. Over time, Cameron's medical trauma began to increase, and he became more and more withdrawn. His brother, Emerson, also started to become annoyed that "everything was about Cameron."

In an effort to decrease Cameron's medical trauma and help the entire family start to return to a better place, Cameron's parents decide to try to get things back into a routine. They decide that they need to set consistent expectations of Cameron. They ask to work with Cameron's favorite physical therapist whenever possible. They schedule his physical therapy at the same time each week and have him do his exercises at the same time every day. Cameron's parents encourage him to think about his exercises like training for sports. They reinstate family dinners and create a set homework time. While the family is not able to fully control the pace of Cameron's recovery, they find that setting up routines and consistent expectations helps decrease stress and fighting.

QUESTIONS TO ASK YOURSELF

- How do I respond when there are changes in my child's medical condition or treatment plan?
- How does my child respond to changes in their medical condition or treatment?
- What does my family already do to help promote consistency?

ACTION STEPS

- In your C.O.A.C.H. notebook, make a list of aspects of your child's medical care that you *can* control.
- Make a list of aspects of your child's medical care that you *can't* control.
- Pick one part of your child's care and create a consistent routine around it.

17

Behavior Charts

Not Bribing, Rewarding

Call it what you will. Incentives are what get people to work harder.

—Nikita Khrushchev

What is love except another name for the use of positive reinforcement?

—B. F. Skinner

Why should I reward my child for doing what they should be doing in the first place? This is a very common question. We do want our children to become self-motivated human beings and to cooperate because they "should." But if something is challenging for your child, they may need extra incentives or support to be able to achieve it. Ask yourself this: Would you go to work if you didn't get paid even if you are doing awesome things at work? Maybe . . . or maybe not. What about doing extra hard assignments at work? Things you are afraid of? Things that are painful? Things that are stressful? For no pay? For how long? We can take this into account when we think about the types of situations we want to help our child with or what behaviors we want to encourage with rewards.

What's the difference between a bribe and a reward? Generally speaking, when you use a behavior chart with a reward built in, you have thought about and communicated expectations ahead of time. You have planned it. You are working to prevent stress and frustration both in your child and yourself. You are using the reward to help your child learn a new skill or complete something that is tough for them. It is *proactive.*

Bribes, on the other hand, we tend to use more out of desperation. We tend to bribe when things are not going well. They are often *reactive*. For example, if you are fighting with your child about getting a shot and can't get them to sit still, you might start making promises to try to calm them down (e.g., we will get a cookie after this; you can play your video game for an extra hour). This falls more into the bribe category. Often parents are already frustrated, and children may already be upset. The bribe isn't tied closely to a behavior that you are trying to fix—you are more just trying to survive. It is less about skill building and more about getting through the moment. Sometimes a well-placed bribe is a lifesaver (and most of the parents we know occasionally toss a bribe into the mix, including us!), but that's not what we are talking about here.

Rewards are proactive.
Bribes are reactive.

Reward systems work. Research has shown us that setting up clear reward plans can help children achieve goals.[1] When should you consider a reward chart? Consider times you find yourself repeating over and over what your child needs to do:

> "Get your shoes on so we can go to the doctor." "Get your shoes on or we are going to be late." "Get your shoes on!" "Get your shoes on *now* or you are going to have a time-out!"
>
> "Let Dr. Smith check your ears." "Please come sit down for Dr. Smith." "I need you to sit for Dr. Smith so she can see if you need medicine." "If you don't let Dr. Smith check you *right now,* there will be no TV tonight."

Reward charts can help to interrupt this frustrating cycle and set up a system in which you and your child are working together to achieve your goals, though the goals may be different: your goal may be for your child to cooperate so an appointment is less stressful for everyone and goes more smoothly. Your child's goal may be to earn their reward, but the outcome is that the behavior you need to happen *happens.*

TIPS FOR CREATING REWARD CHARTS

1. **Choose one behavior or goal at a time.** Sometimes when things are feeling stressful or challenging with a child, parents can rattle off a full list of behavior changes they'd like their child to make. It can be hard to narrow it down to start small. You may want to start with either (a) the behavior that you are most likely to be able to change or (b) the behavior that is creating the most stress for your child or you.
2. **Set clear expectations.** Take time to ensure your child understands their new job or expectation. Imagine that you are at work and your boss has set a new goal for you but doesn't tell you what it is or doesn't explain it clearly. This can be incredibly frustrating. Similarly, children can become frustrated when they do not know or understand what is expected of them.
3. **Set goals low, and grow slowly over time.** When you first set up a reward chart, make sure your child can achieve your expectations. When your child earns their reward, you both win. The goal is that your child will begin to engage in the behavior over time, even without the reward. This allows you to build in new goals. If your child begins easily achieving their goals, then you can praise them for it and make a new goal.
4. **Set reasonable rewards.** Think about your child and your family. Different children respond to different types of rewards. For example, some children may enjoy choosing a favorite meal, while others might prefer choosing a game to play with the family. Teenagers may prefer to earn screen time, time with friends, or money. Some parents choose to use tangible rewards such as stickers or toys. Some parents buy or make a treasure chest with a range of rewards the child can choose from. Be sure to choose a reward that works for you as a parent as well.
5. **Consider your child's age and cognitive ability.** Can your child understand earning points, stickers, or tokens to turn in for a prize later? Or do they need an immediate reward?
6. **Do it together.** Once you have decided what goal you are setting and have an idea of a reward, you may want to sit down with your child and create the chart together. This can help your child get excited about the rewards or become more comfortable with the new plan.

7. **Behavior charts often need to be modified over time.** Sometimes the rewards lose their effect and need to be adjusted as well.

Daniel's Rewards

We learned earlier that Daniel has struggled with his infusion appointments—both before and during his infusions. His grandparents try several strategies. They start medical play at home and talk with his medical team at the hospital about reward charts. When they first start his rewards, they recognize that they can't go from what they currently would describe as a disaster (Daniel kicking, screaming, and refusing to get in the car to go to the hospital; refusing to get out of the car at the hospital; physically fighting his port access; and screaming at the nurses and doctors throughout the entire appointment) to an easy appointment.

They work with the medical team to build rewards into different phases of the appointment as well as create their own chart. Daniel decorates his chart and gets excited about his rewards. Daniel is obsessed with cars, so they choose car stickers and matchbox cars as their rewards. For every five stickers Daniel earns, he gets to choose a matchbox car out of a treasure chest at home. The hospital also provides a matchbox car that Daniel can earn during each infusion once he completes his sticker chart for the day.

In the beginning, Daniel's behaviors are far from perfect. But slowly, over time, he starts to focus more on the rewards he is earning, and his fears about the hospital and infusions start to improve. Table 17.1 shows the first reward chart Daniel's grandparents used.

Table 17.1. Daniel's First Reward Chart

Eats breakfast: No yelling allowed	Gets in car: Daniel can cry, but no hitting or kicking allowed	Gets out of car to go into hospital: Daniel can cry, but no hitting or kicking allowed	Lets nurse take vitals without needing to be held down: Crying allowed	Gets IV started: No kicking or hitting; okay to need help from family/nurses; okay to cry	Watches show quietly for two minutes during infusion; can get sticker every two minutes

5 stickers = 1 matchbox car
Note that 100 percent is not required to achieve his reward.
As Daniel's behaviors improve, his grandparents adjust his chart, increasing expectations.

QUESTIONS TO ASK YOURSELF

- Is my child struggling with any behaviors that I might be able to improve using a reward chart?
- What types of rewards excite my child the most?

ACTION STEPS

- In your C.O.A.C.H. notebook, make a list of things that you could use as rewards for your child.
- Choose one behavior that your child needs extra help with. Use this behavior to create a chart for them.

18

Additional Visual Supports

Creative Preparation

Nothing is particularly hard if you divide it into small jobs.

—Henry Ford

Different children learn in different ways. We can talk and have children listen (auditory), provide handouts and use whiteboards (visual), and engage children in hands-on problem solving (tactile). Children who are experiencing medical trauma may vary in how they best learn and experience support. Visual supports, such as visual schedules and teaching stories, are tools you can use with your child to help them prepare for upcoming medical events such as appointments, vaccines, or procedures. Visual supports can be particularly helpful for children who are very young or who have cognitive impairments. However, visual schedules and teaching stories can be helpful for most children in daily life.

One of the sources of stress in everyday life, but in particular with medical trauma, is uncertainty. Children who have experienced trauma or very stressful medical situations can develop fears that these events will happen again. Children are sometimes not even aware they have these fears or are unable to describe them.

Visual supports can help children know what to expect. More than just telling your child what will happen, visual supports are something you can point to if your child forgets or starts to panic.

Visual supports can also be used to break down otherwise stressful or scary events into smaller parts that help the child manage their expectations.

Visual supports are not unique to managing medical trauma. They are often used to support daily functioning and help children with special needs, such as autism, learn new skills.[1,2] Visual supports reduce uncertainty and break down your adult "big picture" world into pieces your child's brain can manage.

Visual supports reduce uncertainty and break down your adult "big picture" world into pieces your child's brain can manage.

This chapter describes how to create effective visual schedules and teaching stories, physically or with particular electronic tools (such as apps or websites), and describes options for how to use them to support a medically involved child.

VISUAL SCHEDULES

What are visual schedules? Simply put, visual schedules are a series of images arranged in a sequence to represent upcoming activities in a child's day. The images can be actual photographs, representative images, line drawings, symbols, text, or other visual formats—the point is to use something symbolic that the child can associate with that event or activity.

There are a number of different types of visual schedules, such as daily schedules and task-focused schedules. The most effective schedules provide some way to indicate that the activity is complete, such as moving the images from the schedule column to the completed column. Similar principles are used with chore charts, school schedules, and even checklists for adults.

Daily visual schedules include the day's major activities and can help a child learn a routine or see that today is different than their typical day. Let's say that your young child has an upcoming surgery. Maybe you're already using some type of schedule to represent their typical day. You could create a visual schedule for the surgery day, retaining some of the familiar, comforting activities both before and after the surgery.

Task-focused visual schedules break down a particular event or skill into smaller steps. For example, a task-focused visual schedule

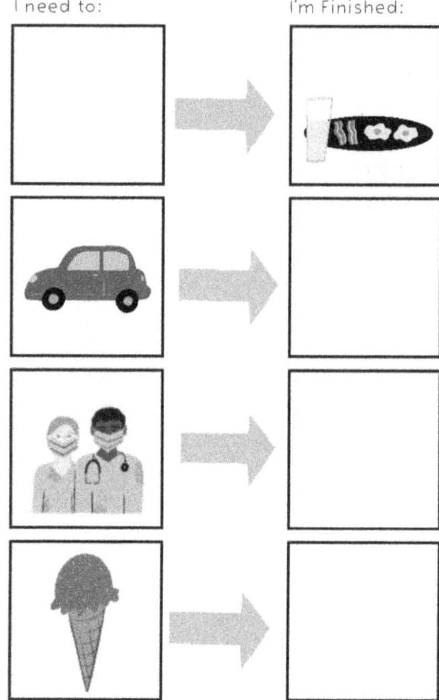

Figure 18.1. Example of a Visual Schedule

can walk a child through the steps of a weekly medical appointment, such as physical therapy or an infusion, or even break down the steps of new skills, such as washing hands or tying shoes. The idea is the same—take what might otherwise feel overwhelming to your child and break it into bite-sized pieces.

Let's jump into the nuts and bolts of creating a visual schedule. Here are some steps:

1. Identify the routine, activity, or skill that you want to target (daily, task, activity).
2. Break it down into smaller steps that your child can understand. Use the C.O.A.C.H. process to collect information about what those steps look like when you're targeting medical procedures. You may need to ask the medical team for more information.

3. Decide what format to use if you're using images. Do you want to use actual photographs? Do you want to find cartoon pictures? Do you want to have your child draw pictures?
4. Figure out how you want to show that part of the activity is completed. For example, do you want to use Velcro or magnets to attach the pictures to a board so you can move the item to a "done" space on the board? Maybe your older child would respond better to a wipeable checklist?
5. Create the schedule physically or digitally. We'll talk more about that in the next section.
6. Teach your child how to use the schedule by talking through it and working with them. Over time, you can reduce your support, and your child will likely feel a sense of accomplishment as they use their schedule.
7. Reinforce their success with praise or a reward.

TEACHING STORIES

Similar to a visual schedule, teaching stories are also intended to create familiarity and increase certainty. They help your child know what to expect. Instead of a simple sequence of visual events, teaching stories take a particular experience and put it into a visual story format using characters similar to the intended audience. For your child, you might create a story about a child going to the doctor's office or to the hospital that you can print and read to your child. Or you can create it digitally in an app or a program. Like visual schedules, teaching stories are common outside of the medical context, and there are many resources to support their use.

To find a story about a specific medical event your child is facing, you may want to search the web using the following key terms: the name of the medical event, "teaching story," "social story," and/or "social skill story." If you can't find an appropriate story and like to write, you might consider creating a teaching story for your child about their specific medical challenges.

PHYSICAL OR DIGITAL?

In a world where so much that was once physical and tactile—books, letters, to-do lists—is now capable of going digital, we often face the question, physical or digital? When it comes to visual supports (or anything really), the answer revolves around utility. Which format will best help you accomplish your goal?

In the case of visual supports, you need to ask yourself a few questions:

1. How does my child learn best?
2. Which format allows my child to access the support and use it as independently as possible?
3. Would it be helpful for my child to have the support with them in more than one place? If so, which format is most easily transported (to the doctor, the hospital, school, etc.)?

You might decide that one format is the best for all your child's visual supports or teaching stories. Or it might be that certain supports work best on your child's tablet or your phone and some are better printed out or on a poster.

For physical visual supports, there are a few options. Especially for visual supports that will be used regularly (e.g., a daily schedule or regular hospital visits), you can print out individual images that might be needed, laminate them, put Velcro on the back, and then create a schedule for a particular visit.

For example, you might have images of different doctors or nurses your child might see (or generic images of medical providers), images of the types of medical equipment that might be used (hospital bed, stethoscope, shot, anesthesia mask), or locations (doctor's office, hospital). You can create a schedule using a single laminated paper with two vertical strips of Velcro—the left being for the upcoming activities and the right for completed activities. So for a particular medical visit, you order the images down the left strip in the order they will occur, then your child moves them to the right strip as each activity is completed.

Another option for visual supports is to create a similar schedule within a notebook that makes it easier for your child to carry with them. As each activity is completed, they move the image to the next page. Extra images (especially for visits that might have unexpected activities but for which it would be helpful to quickly prep your child) can be stored in an envelope or on extra Velcro strips in the back of the notebook.

There are also products that you can purchase that put all of this together for you (some products are listed below), but you may find that the images you need for medical purposes are not always included. You may have to take photos or find other images online, such as from one of the resources listed below.

For task-focused visual schedules or teaching stories in which the same steps happen each time, you can create the sequence or story online or on your computer and then print it out. Laminating the sheet or story is also helpful if it will be used repeatedly, such as with a regular medical procedure or appointment.

There are also websites that offer stock images, templates, and apps for building printable schedules:

- ABA Educational Resources: www.abaresources.com/free-downloads (picture schedules and social stories)
- ConnectAbility: connectability.ca/visuals-engine (create schedules and stories to print; includes stock images and the ability to upload your own)
- Do2Learn: do2learn.com (a paid app to create visual supports including schedules and behavior charts; website also offers free picture cards, including medical ones, and other resources)
- SchKIDules: www.schkidules.com (magnetic and Velcro visual schedules for purchase; more information on visual supports)
- Geneva Centre for Autism: www.autism.net/resources/visual-gallery (sample visual schedules, templates, and stock images)
- LessonPix: lessonpix.com (low-cost membership-based site to create visual supports)

If you've concluded that digital is the best course for one or more of your child's visual supports, there are a variety of options. It can be as simple as dropping images into a notes, photos, or word processing app on your phone or your child's tablet or downloading specific apps that will make the process easier and save each support for you.

Here are some apps that offer digital solutions for visual supports:

- First Then Visual Schedule HD
- Visual Schedule Planner
- Scene Speak

- Choiceworks
- Routine Factory

New apps are being developed all the time, so to stay up to date on new digital visual supports, search "visual schedule," "visual support," or "social story" in your app store.

Your local health care provider or institution might also offer visual supports such as videos or printables on their website. This is a question that you can ask as you collect information in your C.O.A.C.H. process. For example, on their website, Children's National Hospital in Washington, DC, offers a video on coming to the hospital and printable visual supports including visual schedules and teaching stories for Coronavirus, EEGs, IVs, blood draws, and clinic visits.[3]

Jin's Stories and Schedule

Jin, who we learned was recently diagnosed with type 1 diabetes, is struggling with all the additional demands put on her in order to maintain her blood sugar, especially because she is so young and doesn't really understand why she has to do these things.

At Jin's well visit, Jin's pediatrician tells Amy about a story she saw online that teaches kids about their diabetes. At home, Amy searches online and finds several teaching stories that explain diabetes in very simple terms. They also tell stories about children like Jin who are getting their fingers poked and who take medicine.

Even as Jin starts to understand a little more about her condition, Amy still feels like she is constantly calculating carbs or poking Jin's finger for blood or giving insulin. It has become a little more routine, but there are days when Jin's blood sugar varies so much that it is overwhelming for both of them.

One of Jin's teachers at school suggests creating a visual schedule for her. Her teacher notes that it might help Jin understand exactly when she gets to do things she enjoys and when she might need to go to the nurse or otherwise have her blood sugar checked at home. The teacher works with the nurse to create a visual schedule for school and sends a copy home for Amy to talk about with Jin. She even offers to help create one for home.

Amy decides to learn more about visual schedules and makes one for home herself. She thinks about Jin's morning tasks: getting dressed, brushing teeth, eating breakfast, grabbing her backpack, in addition to taking care of her diabetes. At first, Amy just lists the tasks in chronological order and prints it for Jin to follow. Eventually, Amy prints pictures representing each activity and makes a board where Jin can move the tasks from one column to the other as she completes them. Amy makes one for the afternoon as well. She also sprinkles in one or two activities that Jin really enjoys, usually right after the diabetes tasks, so Jin knows something enjoyable is coming up.

QUESTIONS TO ASK YOURSELF

- Does my child ask questions and seem nervous about what's going to happen with specific appointments or procedures?
- Which of my child's routines or medical events would be appropriate for a visual schedule?
- Does my child learn best on a physical or digital platform?

ACTION STEPS

- Decide if your child could benefit from a visual schedule. If so, choose one to start with.
- Visit one of the websites featured in this chapter (or search for others) to learn more about creating and using visual supports.
- Follow the steps above to create a daily or task-focused visual schedule for your child's most pressing medical (or other) need.

19

Desensitization

Let's Get Used to It

> You can't be that kid standing at the top of the waterslide, overthinking it. You have to go down the chute.
>
> —Tina Fey

Desensitization is normally understood as a process of exposing someone to a potentially anxiety-inducing situation in small doses, allowing them to slowly and calmly master their fear. Think of it like allergy shots—a little bit over time helps your body tolerate something that might otherwise cause a strong negative reaction.

The challenge in the case of children who have chronic illness or who require many medical interventions is that there are few opportunities to desensitize a child to the medical world. Often it just feels like *more* medical involvement. This chapter describes small changes that you can make and actions you can take to help your child get used to some of the challenging medical scenarios.

Therapists sometimes engage in a process called systematic desensitization, which is most appropriate for significant levels of anxiety. Depending on your child's level of fear or anxiety, it may be helpful to work with a therapist. Unlike systematic desensitization, which requires a trained mental health professional, the suggestions in this book involve small changes you can make in your child's daily life that can help them get used to medical care.

FACING MEDICAL FEARS

If your child exhibits fear of medical interventions, your instinct might be to avoid anything medical unless it's required. You might avoid talking about doctors, turn off the television when a medical show comes on, or take the long way around to avoid driving by the hospital on the way to a friend's house. This is a natural and very common reaction. Our minds and bodies instinctively want to avoid people and places that cause fear or other negative emotions. This is called conditioned fear.

Avoiding things we fear is a natural and common reaction, but avoidance gives fear power.

Typically what happens when we fully avoid our fear is that we give it more power and try to avoid it even more. Desensitization can help us to conquer these types of fears and take more control of our body's reactions.

So what are some small steps you can take in desensitizing your child to medical trauma?

Step 1: Stop avoiding your child's natural exposure to medical situations, if you are doing that. Go about your daily life, and if there happen to be medical topics, medical locations, or medical personnel involved, let your child see it. Note: This doesn't apply to very scary or potentially traumatic conversations or medical shows. Use your judgment about what is appropriate for your child. If you are unsure, ask their medical team for advice.

Step 2: Initiate some intentional exposure. This could start with just talking about medical providers, places, or procedures with your child. Depending on your child's age, maybe you watch a movie or television show that has a medical aspect to it. As mentioned before, choose your shows carefully. Notice your child's response. Ask questions about what they think. Being exposed to health care outside of their own experience can help children see it in the context of their life and the lives of others and help them feel less alone.

Step 3: Start talking more specifically about your child's own medical experiences. Listen to what your child has to say. Try not to avoid the hard conversations. Ask for help from your child's medical team if you need it.

Step 4: Consider medical play, if appropriate for your child's age and development. As we'll discuss more in the next chapter, medical play is another form of desensitization. Bringing home extra (safe) hospital supplies or purchasing some yourself will allow you to walk your child through some of their medical experiences surrounded by the safety and comfort of your home and family.

Step 5: Allow the medical play to translate to when your child is actually at a medical appointment. If it seems like it might be helpful to your child, let the provider know that you'd like time for your child to examine the medical devices themselves, such as the stethoscope or pulse oximeter, before the devices are used on them. Maybe your child wants to listen to your heart or check your oxygen first. Many pediatric providers are used to engaging in these back-and-forth exchanges with children.

As mentioned previously, showing your child medical circumstances that are not about them can be helpful. One way to do this is to visit medical locations for some other purpose. Do you have to pick something up? Is there someone to visit at the hospital? Is there a special event happening there that you could attend with your child? If every time they show up at a doctor's office or hospital scary and painful things happen to them, it will be hard to break their fear cycle. If you pepper in casual and even fun appearances, your child can become less conditioned to be afraid of medical care.

NORMALIZATION

Another aspect of desensitization is to normalize medical interventions as much as possible. This includes how you talk about appointments, procedures, and your child's other interactions with the health care system. It can be helpful to talk to your child about other children with their same medical condition. Sometimes you can find books to read or support groups so that your child learns that they are not alone.

As we discussed in the previous chapter about visual supports, try to surround medical interactions with other routine parts of your child's life. Balance keeping things consistent with your daily routine before and after appointments with having some rewards. When you do visit the hospital or doctor's office, take along activities that your child routinely enjoys—books, videos, games. If you have time, work in some lunch at the hospital cafeteria (and maybe some ice cream!) and a walk outside if the weather is nice. As much as possible, make medical appointments seem just a part of everyday life instead of big, mean, scary events.

Work with your child to normalize their medical care so that they don't feel like they have to hide it from others. You can tell your child that it is okay to take medicines or shots or do treatments (as appropriate) in front of others. If this is new for your child, consider starting with a close family member or friend, and plan it with them ahead of time. You may want to prepare the family member or friend in advance so they are comfortable as well. But if your child is not ready for this and wants to do their treatments privately, support that choice. Another option might be for you to ask other family members to take a medication or do a treatment in front of your child so that they start to see others' comfort with this.

Try to surround medical interactions with other routine parts of your child's life.

MUSCLE MEMORY

One desensitization technique is to use muscle memory. Muscle memory involves repeating a motor task over time so that eventually it can be performed without conscious effort. With muscle memory, your child doesn't have to pay as much attention to it, so they can instead distract themselves.

Consider whether there are specific movements necessary for regular medical interventions that your child has. One example is where a child needs to hold their arms up and arch their back for a nurse to access a port-a-cath. Practicing these positions at home before they are required in a time-sensitive situation can help your child get comfortable with them. Then, when they are needed in a medical atmosphere, your child (with or without your help) is able to perform them without as much conscious effort. They pay less attention to the movement itself as a source of anxiety. If it is practiced over time, outside of a medical context, their minds also tend to associate it less with traumatic events, and overall anxiety at the event can potentially be reduced.

Cameron and the Car

Throughout his recovery, Cameron has avoided the car. He is slow to get ready and quiet while he rides. It is such a problem that Zoe and Preston end up doing errands by themselves and mostly staying home on the weekends. As Zoe feels them all beginning to engage in these avoidance behaviors alongside Cameron, she decides to use the C.O.A.C.H. process to try to deal with this issue.

Zoe begins by *collecting* information. Since Cameron won't talk to her, she reads about how injuries can affect a teenager's emotional health over time. She asks his therapist for more information about how to support Cameron with his fear of the car.

She *observes* his behaviors, noticing that he is no longer going to friends' homes if it requires him to ride in the car. She realizes that they are all starting to avoid extra car rides. She also notices that Cameron gets ready for the day with no problems if the day doesn't include medical appointments or car rides.

She *asks* Cameron if he has any ideas about how to make the mornings go better and if his medical appointments are difficult for him. She also calls the medical team to see if his current behaviors are normal. Zoe asks the medical team for suggestions about how to get Cameron more comfortable in the car, and she asks the school and her work for flexible arrival times for the next month.

Zoe then *chooses* to try a form of desensitization by having Cameron practice riding in the car on the weekends, when there is no time pressure. She suggests that they grab doughnuts for the family or take their dog Brody to the dog park. Zoe also thinks about timing and starts waking Cameron up an hour earlier to get ready for school so there won't be so much pressure. She also creates a reward chart to encourage Cameron to get into the car by a certain time during the week.

While Zoe's strategies take some time to start working and don't solve the entire challenge with Cameron, she feels better that she is able to *help* him.

QUESTIONS TO ASK YOURSELF

- Am I or is my child avoiding situations involving medical people, places, or circumstances?
- What medical interactions seem to cause my child the most anxiety?
- How can I incorporate one or more of the desensitization techniques into my child's daily life?

ACTION STEPS

- Plan and engage in one conversation with your child about medical care (theirs or someone else's—real or fictional, such as a situation portrayed in a television show).
- Plan and implement one interaction involving your child with the medical world that does not involve your child's own medical care.

20

Medical Play

Children Learn through Play

Play gives children a chance to practice what they are learning.

—Fred Rogers

There is something disarming about play. Your child's imagination, curiosity, and joy combine so that they experience life in a way where they learn, are soothed, and teach, all at the same time.

Play can have a crucial role in preventing and managing medical trauma. It can be an invaluable tool in your arsenal to make medical events tolerable and maybe even fun for your child. While the strategies described in this chapter are most effective for younger children who are still engaging in role playing with figures and toys, they can also be incorporated into medical trauma challenges facing older children and adolescents.

Play can have a crucial role in preventing and managing medical trauma.

Professionals such as child life specialists or hospital-based psychologists are often trained in techniques for medical play therapy. If they are available in your area, reach out to them for help as you consider this strategy for your child. You may not have time to add another medical appointment with them into your child's schedule, but they might be able to stop by when you're already at the hospital or take a phone call to give you some ideas. Or if your child needs extra help, squeezing in that appointment might be worth it.

As we discussed in the previous chapter on desensitization, it can be helpful to bring home extra medical supplies or purchase portable devices that are used in your child's care, such as stethoscopes, pulse oximeters, or anything else your child regularly comes into contact with. If the real items aren't available or appropriate, you can find many pretend medical kits that vary in their realism. Maybe this involves infusion kits, shots, stethoscopes, anesthesia masks, nasal cannulas, or other items. Consider adding any items that your child has or might associate with pain or fear in a medical setting. Also add things that they are comfortable with so they can slowly expand medical play if they need to.

TAKING DESENSITIZATION A STEP FURTHER

While desensitization strategies involve your child becoming familiar with these items, medical play goes a step further and encourages your child to *use* these items themselves. Instead of the patient, they might become the doctor, nurse, or narrator of the story. Or they might request for you or a sibling to play as their doctor.

Maybe your child creates a doctor's office out of your family room, and their stuffed animals visit the same doctor they do. Maybe their dollhouse becomes a hospital with a waiting room, surgery suite, and recovery room. They can become both the medical provider and the patient.

The point is that they regain control over the series of events that are normally happening *to them*. As the American Academy of Pediatrics notes,

> Play allows children to create and explore a world they can master, conquering their fears while practicing adult roles, sometimes in conjunction with other children or adult caregivers. As they master their world, play helps children develop new competencies that lead to enhanced confidence and the resiliency they will need to face future challenges.[1]

When your child feels more like a participant in their own medical care, they will be less fearful.

At first, don't attempt to direct any of the play. Let your child lead the way, and observe or follow them. Pay attention to how they play out various scenarios and what their characters have to say, what they're afraid of, and how they react; this might give you insight into your child's fears and anxieties.

If your child avoids any medical scenarios similar to their own when they are playing, wait until they have become comfortable with medical play. Then possibly suggest that one of their characters is facing a medical challenge described as similar to theirs. The character needs their help. How do they respond?

For older children, rather than "playing," they could write a play or a book about their medical experiences. Follow your child's lead, and let them control the story and characters. If you are concerned about their story or responses, ask your child's doctor for help.

COMMON LANGUAGE

In chapter 15, on communication, we discussed working with your child to develop some common terms for people, places, and things involved in your child's medical care. Medical play can also help you and your child settle on a common language.

Using pretend or extra medical supplies, engaging in playacting as a medical provider, and using play equipment brings life to the conversation. You can observe their natural interactions and let them take the lead in labeling. Try to use short, descriptive terms, ideally one to three words.

CELLIE COPING KITS

One specific product that might support your effort to engage your child in medical play and to teach your child coping strategies is the Cellie Coping Kit, invented by one of the authors of this book, Dr. Marsac. The coping kit includes a stuffed toy named Cellie, coping cards, and a book for caregivers. Each kit has over one hundred tips for dealing with numerous medical-related stressors, such as medical procedures, hospital visits, and feelings of fear and uncertainty. Cellie's zippered mouth is a great place for your child to keep the cards that they are using or to pack small toys for appointments. The cards can provide a platform for communicating with your child about many of the issues discussed in this book, especially in the context of medical play.

The Cellie Coping Kits are designed for children aged six to twelve years and can be used by your child on their own, with you as a parent, or with other trusted adults, in conjunction with your child's medical team or with their child life specialist or a mental health provider. As of the writing of this book, there are kits available focused on children who are dealing with cancer, sickle cell disease, food allergy, injury, and eosinophilic esophagitis. There is also a coping kit for siblings of children with medical conditions. More are in the works. You can find more information about the kits and science behind the kits at www.celliecopingcompany.org.

As you consider how medical play might fit into your efforts to prevent or reduce medical trauma in your child, focus on the important medical events your child has to endure. Think about the medical events or treatments that are repeated frequently. Consider using medical play so they become comfortable with both the process and their own participation.

Nia Loves to Play

Before she was diagnosed with cancer, Nia had an elaborate doll setup in her room. She could play for hours, making up adventures, jobs, and friendships. Maria would peek in and hear character conversations that made her smile.

The medical demands that came with Nia's cancer haven't left a lot of time for playing anymore. And when she does have time, Nia is often tired or seems more sad than normal.

One day when Nia was supposed to go to the hospital for treatment, she simply refused to get out of bed. Maria encouraged, then coaxed, then threatened, then offered a reward using the behavior chart she developed. Nia finally did get in the car, but then at the hospital, everything else was difficult. She yelled at the phlebotomist wanting to draw her blood and hid her arms inside her sweatshirt. This had been brewing for some time, Maria thought. Nia hated getting her blood drawn. When the nurse wrapped the stretchy rubber band around her arm, Maria watched Nia wince. Nia's lip trembled as she looked away from the needle.

Maria wants to find a way to help and thinks, based on what she's learned and observed, that medical play might be worth trying. She asks the nurse if she can have one of the tourniquet bands and some alcohol swabs. She stops by the child life services office and gets some pretend needles/shots to take home.

When they get home, Maria brings the supplies into Nia's doll area. She doesn't say anything other than, "Sometimes dolls get sick too and might need your help, Nia." At first, Nia ignores the supplies. But a few days later, Maria can hear her soothing her favorite doll in the same voice the phlebotomist at the hospital uses: "Now, it's just a tiny poke. One, two . . . there! It's done!" Maria joins her and asks if Nia is ready to take her mom's blood too. Nia wraps the tourniquet around Maria's arm and says, "Here's your squeezy!" Maria makes note of Nia's new term for that part of the procedure. Once she finishes, Nia looks pleased with herself. Before long, Nia is asking everyone who stops by if she can draw their blood.

The next time they go to the hospital, Nia brings her supplies too. Maria takes the nurse aside when they check in to ask if Nia can pretend to take the phlebotomist's blood too. The team readily agrees. The whole process goes much smoother this time, and Nia is proud of how brave and calm she is during the procedure.

QUESTIONS TO ASK YOURSELF

- Have I already seen my child involve medical scenarios in their play?
- Is my child at a developmental level where they enjoy play figures, role playing, writing books or plays, or some other type of play?

ACTION STEPS

- Gather the supplies, toys, or other items that might be appropriate for medical play and encourage your child's imagination.
- In your C.O.A.C.H. notebook, write down the words your child uses to describe medical personnel, supplies, devices, and appointments/procedures.

21

Adapting the Environment

Make Yourself at Home

I don't want to be a product of my environment. I want my environment to be a product of me.

—Jack Nicholson

Close your eyes. Wait—after you read this paragraph, close your eyes. Notice your senses. What do you hear? What are the loud sounds and the more subtle sounds, the hum in the air? What do you smell? Fresh or stale air? A scent? What do you feel on your skin? How does the air around you feel? What taste is in your mouth?

Now open your eyes. What do you see? Besides this book, are you surrounded by busy or calm? Boring or beauty? How do your senses make you feel? Do they make you feel happy or sad? Or bored? Do they make you think of the things you still need to do today or allow you to feel content to finish this book?

Our environment affects how we feel. That is true in general as well as in medical environments. An important study found that the design of health care facilities can actually influence medical outcomes positively or negatively.[1] The report compiled over six hundred studies that linked health care design to outcomes in patient and staff stress and fatigue, patient safety, and overall health care quality.[2]

Research has also shown that we are happier in beautiful surroundings.[3] Disorder in our environment has been linked to negative behaviors and poorer learning in children.[4] Sounds and smells take us back to specific times. All our senses can trigger memories, both good and bad.

Our environment affects how we feel.

Ideally for children, medical and therapy appointments should be surrounded by an atmosphere of calm and fun. Some children's hospitals and doctors' offices are better at this design than others. Parents can create this atmosphere as well.

The following sections provide some questions to ask yourself and potential strategies for modifying your child's medical environment to prevent or reduce their medical traumatic reactions or to simply help them feel calmer.

SENSE OF HEARING

What does your child hear in anticipation of appointments and at the appointments themselves? What is the tone of your voice? Even if your child is too young to understand the terminology or what is actually happening, they still take in a lot of information about how to feel about medical situations from what they hear. Keeping an upbeat or calm tone as opposed to a worried or dreading tone can be helpful.

Laughing and singing on the way to the hospital is one way to engage that sense of hearing in a positive way. Many children's hospitals also offer music therapy, which can be anything from playing an instrument to writing music that expresses emotions.

The report on health care environments mentioned earlier found noise to be one of the challenges related to poorer health outcomes, including lower oxygen saturation, loss of sleep, lower patient satisfaction, and higher stress.[5] Many hospital rooms, and especially intensive care units, are filled with beeping and buzzing and dinging, enough to alter sleep patterns and startle even adults. In many cases, there is not much that parents can do to reduce the overall hospital noise. Keeping doors closed in single rooms can be helpful. Also, having a tablet or smartphone (or borrowing one from the hospital when possible) with which your child can listen to music, watch movies or their favorite television show, or make video calls to family members helps drown out some of the drone of the hospital and provides welcome distraction. Sleep machines, sound machines, or apps (even with headphones for louder environments) can also be helpful for overnight stays. Some hospitals may even have sound machines available; you may need to ask.

SENSE OF SIGHT

You can't control everything your child sees at the doctor's office or the hospital, but you can provide distraction and comfort through the visual aspects of their medical appointments. Are there special movies that your child loves? Special books? It is a great strategy to find items that your child only gets to use during appointment or infusion times or in waiting and pre-op rooms.

What a child sees in the medical environment may also become a focus if they are not distracted. If your child is in the hospital, are there posters or pictures from home that you could put up around the room? Games that you could play? A special lamp you could bring in that reminds your child of their bedroom? Pictures or cards from friends or family to hang up? Maybe even bring a slipcover for that sterile hospital chair to make it feel more like home. If there are curtains in the hospital room, consider opening them to get a view of the outside world.

Light can have an impact on your child's medical experiences. Studies have shown that bright light in medical spaces can help reduce depression and that morning light is twice as effective as evening light.[6] Sunlight in particular has been shown to be associated with lower perceived stress, less pain, and less pain medication used.[7] So if your child is expecting or ends up with a hospital stay, it would be worth it to ask about a room with natural light. Or you can ask if your child can go outside while the sun is out. Of course, if the lights in the room have a dimmer, that often helps when it's naptime or nighttime.

> *Sunlight is associated with lower perceived stress, less pain, and less pain medication used.*

Viewing or being in nature is also associated with reduced stress and anxiety, lower pain, and higher pain tolerance.[8] Connecting a nature experience, whether with a walk before or after an appointment, a nature video, or a hospital garden, could help reduce your child's anxiety and create more positive feelings.

SENSE OF TOUCH

Consider both what your child touches as well as what and how something or someone touches them. Some children have that special blanket or animal, and holding it during stressful appointments and procedures can create a feeling of calmness. A weighted blanket can also be calming for many children (and adults!). Consider bringing your own towels to the hospital and asking if your child can wear their own clothes and pajamas instead of hospital-issued ones.

Your physical interaction with your child may also play a key role. Studies show that parents' touch establishes an infant's feelings of security, brings on positive emotions and smiling, and helps manage children's emotions and distress behaviors.[9] If your child appears stressed, behaviors like stroking, hugging, and holding your child might help reduce that distress.[10]

It can also help to maintain your typical amount of contact during a medical appointment, as you would normally have at home. For example, what kind of physical contact is your child used to at home? Do they often sit in your lap? If so, consider requesting that medical procedures (e.g., needle sticks), where possible, happen with your child in your lap.

Consider animal interactions as well, especially if you already own a pet or your child enjoys animals. Studies indicate that a child's interaction with their own pet during stressful encounters can reduce their perceived stress,[11] although we know it's often not possible to bring your own pet to medical appointments. Many hospitals do have pet therapy programs, and especially among patients who have a pet themselves, studies have shown that just petting an animal can lower your heart rate.[12]

SENSE OF TASTE

Having your child's favorite snacks and drinks on hand, as we've mentioned in other chapters, can make the difference between a smooth afternoon and a meltdown. A little lunch box especially for medical appointments is handy. You can offer for your child to carry it to give them a sense of ownership and something to look forward to (as long as they aren't preparing for a procedure where they can't eat or drink and might get tempted to sneak a snack!).

Balancing different flavors and textures with their snacks and meals can also provide some sensory stimulation that many children crave. Chewy items, like gummy bears, can be useful when they seem like they are getting overwhelmed.

If you're staying overnight in the hospital, your child's food situation can vary widely depending on their condition and the facility. In some hospitals, you can order from a wide variety of delicious options and even from local restaurants. But if you can't get something that works well for your child in a given situation, consider bringing your own food, calling a friend, or ordering take-out for your child to enjoy their favorite foods if their condition allows it.

SENSE OF SMELL

Most people can describe the strong scents from a hospital or doctor's office—cleaning products, alcohol, or whatever goes into that highly "medical" smell that makes us scrunch our noses. These scents can be especially alarming for a child and can become subconsciously associated with feelings of anxiety around an exam or procedure. When a child walks into a doctor's office or hospital, the smell alone can trigger an automatic anxious response. One strategy to try if your child is struggling with smells is to counteract those smells with ones that your child finds calming and familiar, like their own lotions, certain foods, their blanket, and possibly aromatherapy.

Consider each of your child's senses as you prepare for your child's next appointment or hospital stay.

Each of your child's senses tells them something about the environment they are in. A sense can communicate safety or danger, joy or sadness, stress or calm. You can take small, deliberate steps to adapt the environment to your child's needs the next time you expect an appointment or even if you unexpectedly end up with a hospital stay. Using the C.O.A.C.H. process, begin to observe how your child reacts based on input to each of their senses.

Cameron's and Zoe's Senses

For the first month after Cameron was released from the hospital, his rehab appointments were at a hospital-based rehab program. For these appointments, they parked in the same hospital parking lot that they had used when Cameron was in the hospital. Zoe noticed that Cameron became quieter as they approached the hospital. On their way to physical therapy in the rehab program, they passed the central area of the hospital. Zoe could smell the cafeteria and remembered long nights from Cameron's initial surgery and recovery.

Coming back to the hospital for rehab several times a week brought back lots of memories for both Cameron and Zoe. Zoe asked Cameron what he was thinking about as they proceeded quietly to the rehab wing, but Cameron didn't respond. Zoe suspected that maybe Cameron was having medical trauma reactions, but she wasn't sure if he would bounce back on his own.

Zoe decides to try to change Cameron's experiences of the environment. She starts scheduling his appointments later in the day, when there are fewer people in the rehab center, so it is quieter overall. She asks Cameron for his favorite music, both songs that help him feel calm and songs that help him get pumped up. She creates several playlists for him to choose from to listen to on the car ride and on their way from the car to the rehab program. She asks his physical therapist if he can choose his own music during therapy to have something to focus on other than being in the hospital. She starts bringing strongly flavored coffee for herself to drink as they come into the building, since the food smells are triggering her own emotions. Zoe also asks Cameron's doctors not to stop by unexpectedly, because although they are trying to be supportive, Cameron seems to do more poorly when he has more people from the medical team present.

It isn't easy, but the strategies Zoe puts in place help a bit and get Cameron through his required rehab.

QUESTIONS TO ASK YOURSELF

- Which of my child's senses seems most bothered by a particular medical environment? Which of my senses?

- What are three things I could bring from home to make a medical appointment or hospital stay more comfortable?
- How can I use my own voice and physical interaction with my child to support them?

ACTION STEPS

- In your C.O.A.C.H. notebook, describe the environment of your child's last medical visit according to each of their senses.
- Make a note of one change you could make for each sense to help reduce your child's stress response.

22

Timing

6:00 a.m. or 6:00 p.m.?

Timing is everything.

—Unknown

For kids with medical challenges, timing isn't necessarily everything, but it can be powerful. There are many parts of medical treatment and medical conditions that parents cannot control, including many aspects of timing. For example, when your child gets sick or when the medical team does rounds at the hospital is out of a parent's control. Parents may not have control over recommended medication schedules or when medical care is available (i.e., sometimes parents have to take what is available when scheduling an appointment), but parents can control the timing of some aspects of medical care. Here are a few timing concepts to consider:

1. **Time of year/holidays:** Sometimes we have options about when to start new medications, go into the hospital, or schedule a procedure. If you have a choice, think about the big picture for your family. Are there holiday traditions that you don't want your child to miss? Or would it be easier to schedule procedures over the holidays when your child is off school and you are off work? Would you rather have your child adjust to a new medication when they are out of school? Or would you

rather not have to manage potential new side effects during a school holiday? Plan what is best for your entire family.

2. **Time of day:** Does your child bounce out of bed in the morning ready to leap into the day? Or do they tend to be more of a night owl? This may be something to consider when scheduling appointments or requiring your child to participate in medical care at the hospital. If you child likes to sleep later, consider scheduling appointments later in the day when possible. If your child is in the hospital and likes to sleep in, ask your medical team to try to schedule medications and therapies as late as possible. Sometimes your doctor can shift medication plans by a couple of hours without a problem—this isn't always possible, but it doesn't hurt to ask.
3. **Anticipatory anxiety:** Does your child become anxious or dread going to medical appointments? If so, you may want to consider taking the first appointment of the day to get it over with.
4. **Your own schedule:** If you need to take time off work, is it easier to go in late or leave early? Do you need a full day off any time you schedule an appointment? If so, can you do more than one appointment in a day (if your child can manage this)? If you have other children, do you need time in the morning to get them to school? Do you need to be home for them after school? Do you have a hard time getting up and out the door in the morning? Would you rather have a slower start? Or would you rather get the appointment over with first thing in the morning? Think about your own anxiety. In considering timing, make a plan that works best for your child and for you.
5. **The doctor's office:** Is your child's doctor always running late? Is it hard for your child to wait for their appointment? If so, you may want to consider taking the earliest appointment possible or an appointment right after lunch.
6. **Planned special events:** Consider any special family or school events. Ask your medical team if it is possible to plan around any special events that you have. Sometimes if your child has a lengthy hospitalization, depending on what your child is being treated for, you may be able to leave and return to the hospital. For example, if your child has missed much of their school year and has something coming up such as a school play or dance, you may be able to take your child to the event and then return

to the hospital. While this can't always work out, there is no harm in asking.

7. **Medication timing:** When your medical team is reviewing medication plans with you, be sure to let them know if it sounds doable. For example, let's say that a medication needs to be taken one hour before your child eats and that your child usually eats at 6:30 a.m. and is on the bus to school by 6:40 a.m. This would require you to get your child up at 5:30 a.m. to take their medication. Is this doable? Is this necessary? In some cases, there might be no choice as it is what's best for your child. In other cases, you may be able to work with the medical team to come up with ideas on how to modify the medication schedule. For example, could your child take it partway through the morning at school rather than first thing in the morning? Some medications also have to be taken frequently. When your medical team tells you the recommended schedule, think through your day. Is there someone who can help your child with a medication four times a day? If it is not possible, tell your medical team and work with them to develop a plan. It is better for them to know of the challenges than for your child to miss medications because the schedule is too hard.

Consider both your child's and your habits and routines as you prepare for your child's next medical event.

Timing for Cameron

We have learned about many of Cameron's struggles along the way, one of which involved avoiding car rides, resulting in being late to school and to medical appointments. When Cameron's mother, Zoe, first started scheduling follow-up appointments, she tried to get them as early as possible so that Cameron would miss less school and so that she would miss less work. However, given that Cameron was already struggling getting into the car and hated getting up early, this was creating lots of family stress. Both of his parents would end up yelling, and he was often late to appointments. Cameron's brother, Emerson, was also often late to school because their parents were trying to get Cameron ready.

As Zoe begins to recognize Cameron's medical trauma symptoms, she realizes that changing their goals for these mornings might also change how these mornings play out. Zoe and Preston come up with a new temporary plan. They decide that until Cameron is better able to manage his anxiety related to medical care, they will try to decrease the morning stress.

Preston and Zoe start taking turns bringing Cameron to medical appointments so that Zoe isn't always the one missing work. Whoever doesn't take Cameron leaves on time with Emerson so he isn't late for school. They start scheduling appointments a bit later in the day to let Cameron sleep a little longer and have more time to get ready without rushing. After a couple of months, as Cameron is doing better with his anxiety, they are able to move the appointments back to earlier in the day.

Nia's Hospital Stay

Earlier in this book we learned that Nia has had a lot of difficulty staying on her time-sensitive medication schedule. Her mother, Maria, worked on this with her and was able to improve this at home. But at a recent hospital stay, Nia refused to take her chemotherapy medications. The medical team worked with her throughout the day and eventually got her to take them, but it took hours, and by the time she took the medications, everyone was frustrated. It happened again the next day.

Nia's mother is exhausted and tired of the fight. She wants this to go better and asks to meet with the medical team to make a new plan. Using the C.O.A.C.H. process, Maria *collects* information about the medications they will be giving Nia.

She *observes* that Nia is having the most difficulty with medications in the morning. Maria notices that nurses are coming in at 7:30 a.m., waking Nia up, and asking her to take medications. Nia is not agreeable. But by 11:00 a.m., after she eats breakfast, Nia is much more cooperative and in a better mood.

Maria *asks* the medical team if they are able to start Nia's medications at 11:00 a.m., after Nia is awake and has had breakfast. The team says they are able to wait until 10:00 a.m. to start medications.

Maria *chooses* to wake Nia up at 9:00 a.m. each day and get her breakfast so that she is ready for her medications by 10:00 a.m.

Maria takes an active role in *helping* Nia have a much better start to the day. While there are still some days when Nia has difficulty waking up and taking her medications, the new schedule is working much better. Maria finds that this new schedule improves the entire hospital stay, decreasing everyone's frustration and allowing Nia to focus more energy on positive activities (such as watching movies and playing games) and less attention and negative energy on medications.

QUESTIONS TO ASK YOURSELF

- What times of day would be best for my child's medical appointments and procedures?
- Could any aspects of my child's medical treatment be improved by a change in timing?

ACTION STEPS

- Review your child's upcoming appointments. Consider modifying appointment times if needed and if possible.

23

Distraction

Squirrel!

Squirrel!

—Doug, from the movie *Up*

Have you seen the Disney movie *Up*? Remember "squirrel"? Throughout the movie, no matter what was happening, whenever the dogs spotted a squirrel, they were completely distracted. This brought humor into the movie but also serves as a great example of how powerful distraction can be.

We can use distraction to help our kids (and ourselves) through medical appointments and procedures. Distraction can help kids feel less pain and be less fearful of medical examinations and procedures.[1] Distraction can also help parents feel less anxious about their child's medical exams and procedures.[2]

Distraction works best when we use it as a short-term solution.

Distraction works best when we use it as a short-term solution. For example, if your child is afraid of needlesticks, it can be helpful for them to focus on something else during the needlestick. For some children, distraction can be as simple as having them blow a pinwheel or sing a song. Other children might prefer playing a video game, watching a show, or listening to a specific music playlist.

Distraction can also be helpful as we prepare for an appointment or procedure. Sometimes our kids' (and our own) anxiety is worse before something happens. For example, let's say your daughter has a surgery scheduled in two weeks that she is already worrying about. You can help her with this anxiety by both preparing her with what to expect and by helping her focus on other things that might reduce her worry. For this type of distraction, you may want to engage your child in activities that require some level of concentration, such as playing a game or doing a puzzle. Worries can be particularly challenging in the nighttime. You might consider using a relaxation app or creating a music playlist for before your child goes to sleep. This can also be helpful as a parent: if you are in the waiting room while your child is undergoing a procedure, reading a book, watching a movie, or doing a word puzzle might help ease your mind.

DISTRACTION TIPS

1. **Plan ahead.** When you think about your child's next appointment, consider if any parts of the appointment may be painful or cause distress. Make a specific plan with your child. If they are able, ask them to help choose what they want to do. If they choose a song, what song? If they want to use a tablet, have them choose exactly what they will do on the tablet.
2. **Bring a new surprise.** For young children, sometimes a new surprise can help. Bubbles and things that spin, move, or light up often work for very short distractions (as long as these are safe for your child).
3. **Bring activities.** When you have to spend time in waiting rooms, bring activities that capture your child's attention: books, art projects, cars, or electronics might be helpful. Things that are new or that you save only for the doctor's office can be especially good for younger children.

DISTRACTION PITFALLS

While distraction can be a very helpful coping strategy, there are a few things to watch out for.

1. **Overstimulation:** Sometimes when we try to distract our child from painful or scary medical procedures, we introduce too much noise or chaos. Imagine you are about to get your blood drawn and are feeling a little nervous. Then imagine that the nurse starts asking you questions to try to distract you, but you begin to feel even more nervous. Then because the nurse sees you are nervous, she grabs another nurse who starts asking you what music you like so that she can put it on her phone. As both of them continue to talk to you, rather than helping, they are making it worse. With the best intentions of helping our child, we often do this with kids, especially those who are anxious or when something isn't going well. The nurse tries to help, Mom tries to help, Dad tries to help, Grandma tries to help, more nurses try to help . . . . What sometimes happens is that we create chaos and a stressful environment while trying to distract rather than using a planned, calm distraction approach.
2. **Choosing the wrong distraction.** Some kids are distracted by pinwheels, some by listening to music, some by telling or listening to a story, some by electronics, and the list goes on. But if you try something and it doesn't work, try something else next time. Or sometimes what used to work doesn't work anymore and you may need a new idea.
3. **Getting distracted from important things.** Some children become experts on refocusing their parents' attention to avoid things. For example, if your child doesn't want to take their medicine, they might try to distract you by asking for hugs first, asking for a book first, asking to call Grandma first, and so on. Allowing your child some control (e.g., Would you like your medicine before or after a hug?) can be helpful. Be careful that they aren't so good at distracting *you* that they are able to avoid their medicine, doctor, procedure, or whatever it is that they need to accomplish.
4. **Sometimes we use distraction too much.** Long-term distraction can turn into avoidance, which may actually prevent us from dealing with our problems. In fact, using too much avoidance when coping with medical trauma has been linked to longer-term trauma symptoms.[3,4] Sometimes we try to distract our child if they are feeling sad about their illness or sad about missing out on something because of their illness. Children need some time

to process their medical challenges and feelings related to them in order to work through them. If we always distract or always avoid feelings or challenges related to illness, these feelings can come out in other ways, such as longer-term anxiety, sadness, meltdowns, or tantrums.

Daniel's Distractions

As we learned earlier in this book, Daniel has Hunter syndrome, which requires weekly infusions at the hospital and lots of medical appointments. Over time, Daniel developed significant medical trauma reactions in which he refused to get in the car for medical appointments and had lots of meltdowns, even when doctors were trying to do basic examinations.

Daniel's grandparents used a combination of strategies to help Daniel cope with and overcome some of his medical trauma reactions. When Daniel needed to have his port accessed and complete lengthy infusions, strategies required planning and keeping a structured, predictable routine with a reward chart.

For some of Daniel's appointments, he just needs to be examined by a doctor. His doctor listens to his lungs; checks his ears, nose, and throat; and feels his stomach. Daniel had become afraid of all doctor appointments because of all the intense treatments he needs. For these more minor appointments, his grandparents are still using a reward system, but they also find that distracting him can be helpful.

Nana and Papa go to a dollar store and load up on cheap light-up toys and stress balls. Before each appointment, Daniel picks a new toy to hold when the doctor comes in. Nana or Papa also set up his tablet with his favorite show playing where he can see it throughout the exam. His doctor learns to quietly enter the room and speak softly to tell Daniel what she is going to do (e.g., I'm going to look in your ears now). She then helps him stay distracted by asking him questions about his show during the exam. Daniel is able to stay calmer during the exam. If a new medical provider comes in, his grandparents explain to the doctor or nurse about what helps Daniel. It doesn't always work perfectly, but it goes much better.

Nana and Papa also work with Daniel at home via medical play and in teaching him about his illness and medical procedures to help him get more comfortable. Over time, Daniel doesn't need as much distraction and starts to handle the "routine" appointments with less support.

QUESTIONS TO ASK YOURSELF

- What types of things help distract my child? Myself?
- Have I used distraction in the past? If so, what went well? What didn't go well?

ACTION STEPS

- In your C.O.A.C.H. notebook, jot down notes about parts of your child's medical care when distraction might be helpful.
- Make a plan for your child's next challenging medical appointment. If there will be something quick, like a blood draw, work with your child to pick out what kind of distraction they want to try.

24

Reinforcement

High Five!

You can't teach children to behave better by making them feel worse. When children feel better, they behave better.

—Pam Leo

Reinforcement is used in order to increase how often a behavior happens. In this book, we will be focusing on positive reinforcement. In positive reinforcement, we add something to help increase a behavior.[1] For example, if you want your child to cooperate with a task like getting ready for a doctor's appointment, you might use verbal reinforcement such as "Thank you for getting dressed without fighting this morning" or "Thank you for getting up when your alarm went off." With kids, even very subtle reinforcement can be powerful: eye contact, smiling, hugging, and laughing are all types of reinforcement.

More tangible types of reinforcement could be actual rewards (see chapter 17 on using reward charts). Rewards can be given either based on a planned schedule or as a surprise. For example, you might tell your child if they are able to take their medicine in ten seconds, they can have a sticker when they are done. Or after your child takes their medication, you could tell them that they did a great job and give them the sticker as an unexpected reward.

We also can unintentionally use positive reinforcement and accidently increase unwanted behaviors in kids. Parental reinforcement is powerful. One of the most common examples of this is when a child does something silly, and parents burst out laughing. This encourages the child to do it again. For example, a child might make up a funny song that is entertaining . . . at first. As the child gets attention from the song, they might sing it again . . . and again . . . and again. And maybe they start to sing the song, which is all about farts and poop, in the grocery store or at school or at dinner. At some point, we may wish we hadn't reinforced the song in the first place.

When your child is singing about farts and poop in the grocery store, you'll wish you hadn't reinforced the song in the first place.

Sometimes even negative attention can serve as reinforcement. Some children will act out to try to get their parents' attention, even if it means being yelled at or getting in trouble. Even the negative attention can increase the likelihood that the child will keep doing the behavior that we don't like.

When we are parenting children with chronic conditions, parental attention can be tricky. There may be times where your child has *all* your attention (e.g., during a hospitalization), but then they have to adjust to normal levels of your attention at home. Or you may have more than one child, and the sibling isn't getting as much attention while you are managing your other child's medical condition.

Sometimes, when children are doing well and doing what we expect, we unintentionally give them less attention. These are times when your children may be looking for any kind of attention and might misbehave to get it. To help counteract accidentally reinforcing behaviors that you don't like, find positive behaviors and load on the praise for those while ignoring or limiting interaction around the negative behaviors.

Reinforcing Behaviors in Nia and Sara

We learned earlier that Nia, an eight-year-old girl who is undergoing treatment for cancer, sometimes struggles with treatments. We also learned that Nia's sister, Sara, has developed symptoms of medical trauma. Maria is recognizing some ways in which she can use positive reinforcement to help support both her girls. She also realizes that she has been unintentionally reinforcing some behaviors in both Nia and Sara.

Maria had already worked with the medical team to *collect* information about which medications were flexible and which had to be taken on a strict time schedule. While changing the medication schedule was helpful, Maria still thought that she may be able to better help Nia through taking her medications.

She *observes* that Nia has more difficulties on days after Maria has been working longer shifts (and consequently has less time with Nia). She notices that Nia is clingier on the days she struggles with medications as well.

Maria *asks* Nia how she feels when Maria has to work long shifts. Nia tells her that she misses her and doesn't get enough time with her. Nia also says that her mother is always on her phone or talking to the doctors when she is there and that she gets bored. Maria considers that some of Nia's acting out about medications might partially be so that her mother will stay with her.

Maria *chooses* to plan and post "special time" for Nia on the calendar. This way Nia will know that she can have her mother's full attention during these times. Maria works to plan extra "special time" before and after long shifts. She also tries to limit the attention that she gives Nia when she won't take medications by letting the nurse take charge of the medications when Nia is in the hospital.

Maria *helps* Nia learn more positive ways to seek attention and takes some of the power away from the medication fight.

Nia's sister, Sara, has been very helpful throughout Nia's treatment. She helps Maria when Nia is fighting about medications, does her schoolwork on her own, and helps out around the house. She tries to be perfect because she doesn't want to burden her mother. However, once Maria learns that Sara is struggling with medical trauma symptoms, she decides that she wants to try to support Sara in a different way.

She *collects* information from Sara's teachers about how Sara is doing and information from the medical team about how to support siblings.

She *observes* that Sara is trying to take care of both Nia and Maria. She also observes in herself that she had been unintentionally reinforcing this. She is so grateful for everything that Sara has been helping with and has been regularly praising Sara for being helpful.

Maria *asks* the school counselor to work with Sara to ensure she has support at school. She asks Sara's teachers for more regular check-ins. She also asks Sara's best friend's mom if Sara can spend more time with them so she'll have a bit more normalcy in her life.

Maria then *chooses* to set aside regular time with Sara. She tells Sara how much she appreciates everything that Sara does to support the family but that it is also okay for her to express her feelings and to need support. When Sara shares feelings—positive or negative—Maria praises her for sharing to reinforce this for Sara.

Maria works hard to *help* Sara start to accept her feelings and to support her coping with Nia's illness.

QUESTIONS TO ASK YOURSELF

- To what kinds of positive reinforcement does my child respond best? How can I use this reinforcement to help my child with their behaviors during medical care?
- Is there anything I do that might be accidentally reinforcing a negative behavior in my child?

ACTION STEPS

- Identify one of your child's behaviors that you would like to change.
- In your C.O.A.C.H. notebook, brainstorm some ideas about types of positive reinforcement that might work for your child.

25

Body Control

Mind-Body Connection

> If you can't fly then run; if you can't run then walk; if you can't walk then crawl, but whatever you do you have to keep moving forward.
>
> —Martin Luther King Jr.

What we think, how we feel, and how our body responds are connected. For example, anxiety, stress, and pain are related.[1,2,3] We described the fear response, or the fight-flight-freeze reaction, in chapter 4. This is how our body responds to very stressful situations: we get ready to fight, run, or freeze in place. This chapter specifically focuses on how to help your child use their own body to manage their fear response.

There are a few steps you can take to help your child gain more control over their body's stress responses. Step one is for you to learn how your child's body responds to fear or stress. Step two is to help your child learn to be aware of their body's responses to fear or stress. Step three is to teach your child strategies to help control their body reactions. Finally, step four is to identify times when your child can use these strategies without your help and when they need your help to support these strategies. In addition to these four steps, there are some general strategies that you can teach your child or use yourself that can help you both stay more relaxed.

RECOGNIZING STRESS RESPONSES

We all react to fears and stress in different ways, but there are some common body responses that are activated with stress. For example, many of us experience tightened muscles, elevated blood pressure, faster breathing, and sweating. Some of these reactions are harder to observe than others.

We all react to fears and stress in different ways.

What might you notice that indicates your child is experiencing fear or stress? Obvious signs might include kicking or fighting a nurse who wants to take a blood sample. Other, less obvious signs could include clenched fists or wringing hands, a tight jaw, headache, rapid breathing, a far-off stare, pacing, or a sudden flurry of activity.

Signs of chronic stress in your body can include stomachaches, decreased appetite, headaches, sleep problems, and strong body reactions to seemingly minor problems.[4]

Take a minute to think about your child. How do they show stress in their body? Consider asking your child how their body feels when something scares them or they are worried. For younger children, it can be helpful to use a picture (maybe the outline of a gingerbread person). With the picture, you can help them label what happens in their belly, heart, legs, and so on when they are afraid. You could also use a favorite doll or stuffed animal. For example, you can ask, "What happens in Giraffe's body when he is scared?" Then you can follow up with "What happens in your body when you are scared?"

RELAXATION STRATEGIES FOR MANAGING STRESS RESPONSES

After you've learned from your child about how their body responds to stressful situations, you can work on ways to help with these reactions. Three common ways to reduce stress are diaphragmatic breathing, visualization, and progressive muscle relaxation.[5]

Diaphragmatic Breathing

Diaphragmatic breathing simply means breathing from your diaphragm. This can be a great technique for kids and parents. There are a few different names for it, such as belly breathing, box breathing, and deep breathing. You can also create your own name for it with your child.

Practice diaphragmatic breathing daily. Bedtime can be a great time to practice. At first, it is best to start practicing when your child is not super stressed. Think of it as a skill you are building. You can try it during stressful situations once you have the hang of it.

Here is one way to teach diaphragmatic breathing:

1. Have your child lie on their back, and place one hand on their upper chest and one on their belly, below their ribs. It might be helpful for younger kids to put a small stuffed animal on their belly that they can watch move up and down with their breath.
2. Ask your child to breathe in slowly through their nose toward their lower belly. The hand on their chest should remain still, but the one on their belly (or the stuffed animal) should move up. Encourage them to make their hand or stuffed animal go as high as possible.
3. Ask your child to exhale slowly through their mouth until all the air is gone. The hand on their belly (or the stuffed animal) should go back down to its original position.
4. Teach your child to breathe out longer than they breathe in. For example, breathe in for a count of four, hold for one, breathe out for a count of five. Adjust the speed of breathing if your child becomes dizzy. Ask your medical team for help if you need it.
5. Repeat for one minute.

Here is a way to teach box breathing. Tell your child to visualize a box. You may want to draw a box on paper or use the one from this book.

1. Inhale: Picture drawing the left-side line of the box going up.
2. Hold: Picture drawing the top line of the box.
3. Exhale: Picture drawing the right-side line going down.
4. Hold: Picture drawing the bottom line of the box.
5. Adjust the speed of breathing if your child becomes dizzy. Ask your medical team for help if you need it.
6. Repeat for one minute.

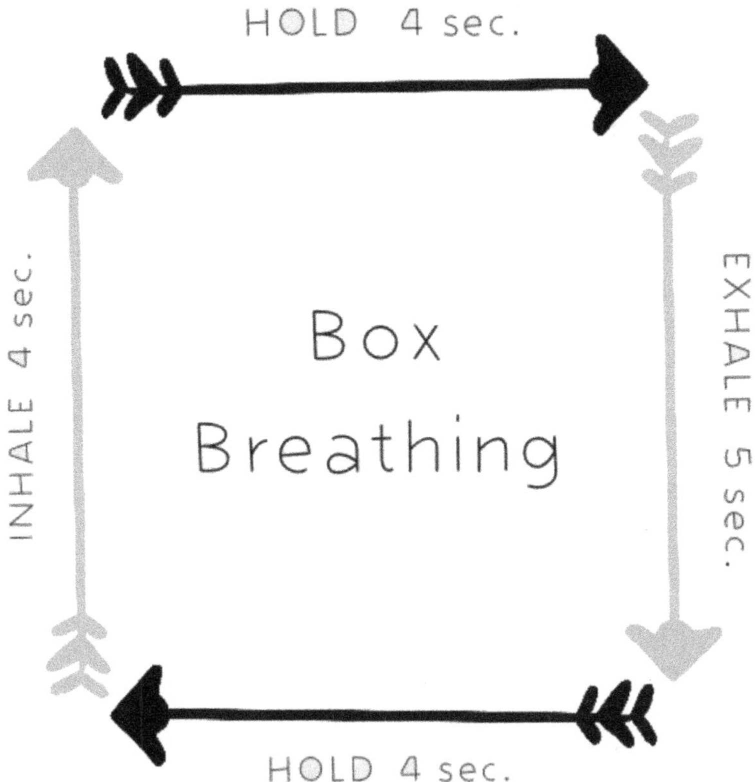

Figure 25.1. Box Breathing

Once you have the basics of breathing down, you can get creative. For example, imagine your child is a butterfly: breathe with the opening and closing of their wings. Or imagine you have just baked fresh cookies. Breathe in to smell the cookies. Breathe out to blow on the cookies to cool them down.

Visualization

Visualization is another technique that can help reduce feelings of stress. This strategy involves using mental imagery, similar to daydreaming. You may have used visualization techniques before to mentally practice before a sports game or race, to rehearse a difficult conversation, or maybe just to remember a pleasant beach from a vacation.

Here is an example of a script to use with your child to help them practice visualization:

Close your eyes.
Imagine a quiet and calm beach.
Just relax here. Breathe slowly and easily. Notice your breath going in and out, in and out. Slow. Easy. It is quiet.
You can feel the sun as it makes your skin warm. Look up and feel it on your face. Watch the fluffy white clouds pass by.
Feel the soft sand under your feet.
The water is warm and just touches your toes. Curl your toes into the sand and feel the water cover them.
Listen to the sound of the waves rise slowly. The water flows over the sand and around your feet. Then it washes back out. Breathe in as the water rises and breathe out as it leaves.
Notice how your breath is calm and even. Slow down your breathing to match the water. Let your muscles relax as you feel the warm sunlight.
Slowly you are relaxing more and more. Your muscles let go of the tension. Your worries are taken out by the waves to the big ocean. Breathe in the calm from the water.
Look at the ocean. It is blue and calm and goes on forever. Its waves wash in and bring you peace, and they take your worries out. The waves keep coming in and keep bringing more peace and calm to you.
Your body is relaxed, and your mind is calm. You can choose to send your worries out with the waves. Feel the warmth of the sun and the water on your feet. Breathe in deeply and remember this moment.
Take in one more deep breath, and bring your mind back to where we are. Bring it back along with the calm and peaceful feelings from the beach.

This is just one example of a script. You can change this one, write a new one, or find more scripts for visualization online. You could choose to visualize a cabin, your child's room, or an open field. Make it your own. Once you begin using visualization with your child, they may express a preference for other places that would calm them too.

Progressive Muscle Relaxation

Another technique for reducing feelings of stress is progressive muscle relaxation. This technique teaches you the difference between relaxed versus tense muscles. You learn how to purposely relax muscles. You might describe it to your child as learning how to transform their muscles from uncooked spaghetti (tense muscles) into cooked spaghetti (relaxed muscles).

Here is an example of a progressive muscle relaxation script. If any part of your body hurts when you tighten it, skip that part:

Lie on the floor or bed.
Take three slow, deep breaths.
Close your eyes.
Tighten your toes and the bottoms of your feet by scrunching them up. Imagine digging your toes into the mud. Hold for five to ten seconds. Relax like a cooked spaghetti noodle.
Tighten your muscles in your legs and feet. Flex your feet to the ceiling. Hold for five to ten seconds. Relax like a cooked spaghetti noodle.
Tighten your muscles in your stomach by sucking it in tight. Hold for five to ten seconds. Relax like a cooked spaghetti noodle.
Tighten your arms and your hands. Raise your arms up to the sky. Imagine that you are squeezing an orange in each hand. Get all the juice out. Hold for five to ten seconds. Relax like a cooked spaghetti noodle.
Tighten your neck and shoulders. Imagine you are a turtle sinking your head into your shell. Hold for five to ten seconds. Relax like a cooked spaghetti noodle.
Tighten your muscles in your face. Imagine a fly on your nose. Scrunch your face up to get the fly off. Hold for five to ten seconds. Relax like a cooked spaghetti noodle.
Now let all those muscles relax and notice the feeling of relaxation.
Take three slow, deep breaths.
Enjoy your time as a cooked spaghetti noodle. Notice your relaxed muscles.

Just like the other strategies in this chapter, you can work with your child to get creative. For example, you could replace the image of an orange with a ball or a lemon. If you make practice into a fun game, this can also help reduce stress.

This is another technique that gets better with practice. It is usually easiest to learn lying down, so you might want to start it at bedtime or in the morning. As your child gets better, they can practice anywhere. They can then use it during medical appointments or other stressful situations.

The techniques from this chapter can be helpful for parents and other family members too. Practicing them together can be good for everyone. After you've practiced them at home, talk about how you might use them in stressful situations at the doctor's office or hospital or even in other areas of life.

SUPPORTING YOUR CHILD DURING EXTREME STRESS RESPONSES

Sometimes children's stress responses become more extreme. This can look like a full-blown tantrum, hysterical crying, or even physical aggression. What do parents do then? These situations can cause significant anxiety and even shame in us as parents, especially if we're out in public. This can be very hard for parents.

If your child has challenges that require the use of physical restraint to keep them safe, talk to your child's medical team. Ask them how to hold your child safely.

If your child has challenges that require the use of physical restraint to keep them safe, talk to your child's medical team. Ask them how to hold your child safely.

While it is ideal to avoid holding children for medical procedures, sometimes it becomes necessary. Children sometimes need help getting the treatment they need. As trauma-informed practices have become more common in health care, the use of restraint has become less common. However, many medical providers feel that some sort of restraint is often unavoidable in younger children, such as those of preschool age, who are more likely to resist medical procedures.[6] This is called "therapeutic holding." If your child needs to be held during a medical procedure and you want to help hold, ask your medical team. If you'd rather have the team hold your child, ask for that. Depending on you and your child, sometimes it works better with you holding and other times it works better if you are supporting in another way.

Think ahead when possible. When is your child most likely to lose their ability to control their stress reactions or body? Have a plan in place for medical appointments. Have a plan in place for the grocery store. Depending on the age and size of your child, you may want to consider having another adult with you when your child is more at risk for an outburst. If so, you also want to plan ahead with the other adult. When you plan ahead, it is easier to help your child with their outburst. A plan can also decrease the intensity of your own emotional response.

Sometimes you may be able to wait out your child's response and let it run its course. This is possible if your child's extreme reaction does not put themselves or others at risk. During medical care, some procedures can be delayed. If you are able to remain calm and give it time, you may have a more successful outcome in the end. We realize that this is much easier to say than to do. It can be very stressful and frustrating when your child is struggling with extreme reactions.

Cameron's Family Learns Relaxation Strategies

Cameron has completed multiple surgeries and had time for the bones to heal. In rehab, Cameron is now working on walking. Zoe has watched Cameron experience random, intense bursts of pain in his legs since surgery and can tell that this new goal makes Cameron highly anxious. Cameron's physical therapist tells him that they are going to start getting up more at his next appointment. Cameron responds by coming up with all kinds of reasons to cancel the next appointment.

Zoe and Preston talk with Cameron's physical therapist about strategies that have been successful for other children. They decide to try some breathing and visualization techniques with Cameron. They learn how to do it themselves before they tell Cameron about it. They hope these strategies will help him relax before these upcoming appointments and give him confidence that he will eventually be back to walking and running. As a family, they sit down together one night after dinner. Zoe teaches diaphragmatic breathing to Cameron. They have all been stressed since the accident. Practicing it together actually benefits everyone.

Preston then asks Cameron what it might feel like for him to walk and run again. Cameron describes how much he misses going for a run in the morning. He says that's what he is most looking forward to. Preston asks Cameron to close his eyes. He describes Cameron getting ready for a run, lacing his shoes, then taking off and feeling the wind, breathing in and out. Zoe can see the look of calm and even joy that comes over Cameron's face as he remembers how much he loves running. When they finish, Cameron is much less nervous about the upcoming appointments. He seems more confident that he can handle the therapy and keep healing. Cameron says he is going to keep visualizing that scene when the pain comes and his muscles hurt from rehab.

QUESTIONS TO ASK YOURSELF

- How often do I slow down and take deep belly breaths? How do I feel when I do?
- What are my child's favorite memories or experiences that might be good for visualization?
- Have I ever used a therapeutic hold for one of my child's medical events? Looking back, is there anything I would now change about that experience?

ACTION STEPS

- Practice diaphragmatic breathing, visualization, and progressive muscle relaxation on your own.
- Pick one of the relaxation strategies from this chapter to try with your child.
- In your C.O.A.C.H. notebook, identify any upcoming medical situations where a therapeutic hold might become necessary. Write down what events might trigger it and how you think it should be implemented. Discuss with your child's medical providers.

26

Switching Strategies

If at First You Don't Succeed, Try Again

> I can't change the direction of the wind, but I can adjust my sails to always reach my destination.
>
> —Jimmy Dean

By now you've probably realized that there isn't one guaranteed way to help your child through medical challenges. Maybe you've tried one strategy, and it didn't help at all. Or two. Or three. It can be tempting to give up and tell yourself that there's nothing you can do to help.

But wait. Not so fast.

Ask yourself these questions first:

1. Have I given the strategy enough time?
2. Is there something I can change to make the strategy better fit my child?
3. Do I need to switch strategies?

Not every strategy will work for every child. Children are unique in age, development, personality, and specific medical challenges. The strategies presented in this book are based in science and expert recommendations, but each strategy may need to be adapted for your child. And some strategies might not be the right ones for your child or family.

If you decide one strategy isn't working, jot down what you tried in your C.O.A.C.H. notebook. Add a note about why you think it didn't work. It may be helpful to keep track of the strategies you are using. A few quick notes about what works and what doesn't may be helpful over time. This can be particularly helpful if you need to ask your child's medical team for guidance. You may want to include notes about any immediate impact on how your child is doing with a particular medical event as well as if you've seen an overall change but are unsure what helped.

Not every strategy will work for every child.

After you try a new strategy, it can sometimes be helpful to talk with your child about how they are doing. You may also want to ask how they like the new strategy. For example, some kids are very excited to see how they are improving when they use a sticker chart for rewards. Others might share that they are mad when they don't get 100 percent of their stickers. Knowing your child's reactions can help you adjust the strategies. In addition, asking your child about these kinds of issues will help them see that you care about their opinions. It allows you to give them some control. These discussions will also show your child that they can openly share their feelings and reactions with you.

QUESTIONS TO ASK YOURSELF

- What am I doing that is working well?
- What strategies have I tried that were not helpful?

ACTION STEPS

- Set aside some time to check in with your child. Consider asking them about some of the strategies you are using. For example, if you are using a visual schedule, you could ask, "Do you like knowing about your day with our picture schedule?" Or if you are using rewards, "What are your favorite rewards that we have used? Do you have ideas for new rewards?"
- In your C.O.A.C.H. notebook, jot down a few ideas from your child.
- In your C.O.A.C.H. notebook, make a note about any strategies you want to change or replace.

Part 5

SPECIAL POPULATIONS

27

Children with Cognitive Impairment

> Children are not things to be molded, but are people to be unfolded.
>
> —Jess Lair

The strategies in this book can be applied to children of all ages and abilities, even though every child is unique. Children differ in physical and emotional strengths and weaknesses, likes and dislikes, fears, intellect, and personality. What is easy for one child can be challenging for another.

For those children with cognitive impairment, we may need to adjust some of our strategies. Intellectual capability often affects how we learn. It also affects our capacity to understand and engage with those around us and with the world. Intellectual or cognitive ability is generally measured by an intelligence quotient or IQ. One hundred is considered an average IQ score, and approximately 68 percent of people have an IQ between 85 and 115.[1] People like Albert Einstein or others with high intellectual capacity might have an IQ of 160, which is at the top of the scale.[2]

COGNITIVE IMPAIRMENT

A child with a cognitive impairment, also known as an intellectual disability, has certain limitations in mental functioning and in skills such as communication, self-help, and social skills. Children with a cognitive impairment will generally learn and develop more slowly than typical children. They may struggle to learn new things and may be unable to learn some concepts or skills. For example, they may take longer to learn to speak, walk, and take care of their personal needs, such as dressing or eating. Some of these children may never be able to understand subjects like geometry or biology.

However, children with cognitive impairment can still be successful and live fulfilling lives. If your child has an intellectual disability, know that this book was designed to help you! We know that children of all abilities can be affected by trauma and can benefit from the strategies in this book. Modifying the strategies to fit your child's abilities and interests will better support them. We also know that every child has unique gifts to offer, and it is worth our investment of time and energy to cultivate these gifts. We will refer to a child with cognitive impairment in this chapter as "your child," because even though it might not apply to your situation, it will apply to many readers of this book.

Children with cognitive impairment can still be successful and live fulfilling lives.

Approximately 1 to 4 percent of children have an intellectual or developmental disability,[3,4] and 13.7 percent of school-aged children, a substantial portion of which have some form of intellectual disability, receive special education services in the United States.[5]

It helps to understand your child's level of functioning in order to choose which tools might be the most appropriate. This can also help you to communicate with medical and other professionals. However, we recognize that often parents are more concerned with how their child's cognitive impairment actually affects them in their day-to-day functioning.

Cognitive impairment is diagnosed through the use of standardized tests of intelligence and adaptive behavior. An IQ of seventy was traditionally considered the threshold for cognitive impairment, with levels of severity defined by specific IQ ranges:

- mild cognitive impairment: IQ of fifty to seventy
- moderate cognitive impairment: IQ of thirty-five to fifty-five

- severe cognitive impairment: IQ of twenty to forty
- profound cognitive impairment: IQ below twenty[6]

However, in more recent years, there has been a recognition that intellectual disability is not defined by IQ alone, and the focus has shifted to functional ability.[7]

Children with mild cognitive impairment may take longer to speak and understand concepts. Many of these children can communicate and take care of themselves. In adulthood, they can often live independently with minimal support. They may need some support during transitions or periods of uncertainty.

Children with moderate cognitive impairment usually have trouble communicating. Although they can do some things on their own, they are probably not self-sufficient and are unlikely to live alone even as adults. Sometimes, with moderate support, such as the support available in group homes, they are able to have more independence.

Children with severe cognitive impairment generally have difficulties with motor function, communication, and learning, and they require daily assistance with self-care activities and safety supervision.

Finally, those with profound cognitive impairment often have limited mobility and are unable to take care of themselves or communicate effectively. They require pervasive support for every aspect of daily living.

If your child has an intellectual disability, they may also have behavioral challenges.[8] These could include things like sleep disturbances, agitation and aggression, and self-injury. Negative behaviors may be associated with an underlying condition, frustration over intellectual or communication challenges, or external factors such as abuse, psychiatric conditions, or some other cause.

ADAPTING THE STRATEGIES

In some ways, adaptations of strategies for children with mild and moderate cognitive impairment might seem similar to those for young children. However, children with cognitive impairment may also have slower processing and behavioral challenges. Thus, they will likely benefit from some unique adaptations. In addition, your child may not understand the reason for their medical care. They might have difficulty understanding their disease or surgeries.

These challenges can add another layer of difficulty if they develop medical trauma reactions.

Using visuals is often helpful for children with cognitive impairment, since reading might be a challenge. Your child can focus more on the concept if they don't have to struggle to read. This can allow them to focus on what is being asked of them. Behavior charts and additional visual supports—using familiar pictures of actual people, places, and things—may work best.

Breaking down tasks into smaller steps can be a particularly helpful learning tool for your child. For example, use a visual schedule with each step of a medical visit as opposed to the entire day. Point out each step, and praise your child after it is completed. This can help to get them excited for the next step and boost their feelings of well-being and confidence.

It will likely take more time to implement a strategy and evaluate whether it is helping if your child has an intellectual disability. Patiently repeating terms or instructions will be important for your child. Taking notes in your C.O.A.C.H. notebook will also help you remember what you observe and remain objective in your assessment.

As you and your child work to find a common language for their medical care, the terms you use will probably need to be shorter and more memorable. Depending on your child's preferences and functional ability, they may not even be descriptive in a meaningful way. Children with moderate to severe cognitive impairment might respond better to terms associated with a color, an action, or a sound. For example, a needlestick might be called "one-two-three" because that's what the nurse says before they insert the needle. A stethoscope might be called "listen" because it's in the provider's ears and you want your child to be quiet for a moment.

It may be helpful for you to model how each new strategy works. You may even want to involve a sibling to model it for your child. You may also need to repeat modeling several times. For example, if you choose to create a visual support for your child, create one for yourself and siblings too. Then you can all show your child how they work. If you create a reward chart, follow the same process. Create one for yourself and reward yourself out loud so your child can see it work. Create one for a sibling, and provide the sibling with rewards as well. In using distraction, you might need to show your child how to blow bubbles and even put your hands over theirs to help them do it.

Working to understand your child's unique strengths, weaknesses, and interests can help you capitalize on which strategies might be most effective and how to adapt them for your child. Following are ways to adapt these strategies for children with cognitive impairment:

- Focus on visual supports, especially if reading is a challenge.
- Break tasks down into smaller steps.
- Take extra time to teach concepts and evaluate the strategies.
- Use short words and phrases to label objects, processes, and concepts based on words your child responds to.
- Repeat instructions.
- Model the tasks yourself or ask a sibling to help.
- Identify and build the strategies around your child's unique strengths, weaknesses, and interests.

COMMUNICATING WITH THE MEDICAL TEAM

It is important that your child's medical team understands your child's unique intellectual and/or behavioral challenges. You know your child best. Medical providers will generally assume that your child has typical abilities unless you say otherwise. Describing your child's challenges and strengths and how those affect medical care will be helpful in their care and can help prevent medical trauma that might come from medical providers expecting more of your child than they are capable of.

Having a short script that you can share with medical providers can prevent miscommunications and help establish a good working relationship with your child's medical team.

Below is a template for a note to share with health care providers about your child with cognitive impairment:

> My child's favorite things are ____ and _____. He has _____ cognitive impairment and behavioral challenges such as ______. He generally functions at a ___-year-old level. He won't understand long descriptions, but he can understand __-step directions. He calls a ______ ______. If you do _____, he might ______, so please let me know ahead of time. I can help explain things to him and encourage him to do what you need if you tell me.

Your child's medical trauma may also look a bit different than what parents might see in a typically developing child. This is especially true if your child doesn't understand or can't communicate their feelings. You might have to be extra aware of the signs and adapt the strategies in unique ways.

Daniel and the New Doctor

When Daniel recently started preschool, Nana and Papa already knew that he took longer to learn new things and was a little behind for his age. Sometimes learning new things, like how to put on his backpack, has taken months for Daniel. When they go to the doctor, he doesn't understand many of the things the doctor says. He just keeps trying to jump off the exam table.

Daniel's pediatrician recently retired. Nana is concerned about finding a new one who can work well with Daniel. She hopes to find a doctor who will be patient enough to take the time Daniel needs to get through medical exams, shots, and other procedures. She reads about local pediatricians online. She asks lots of questions of friends and then of the office staff when she calls to learn more. Finally, she finds Dr. Gerard, who she hopes will be a great fit.

Nana decides to make a teaching story for Daniel about their upcoming visit. She prints a big picture of Dr. Gerard from her website and decides to refer to her as Dr. G to Daniel, since that will be easier for him to remember. She adds photos she previously took of a nurse listening to his heart and one giving him shots. She reads Daniel the short story with the terms she collected in her C.O.A.C.H. notebook. They read the story several times before the next visit.

Daniel's "New Doctor" teaching story:

> Daniel *goes to the doctor*.
> Daniel meets *Dr. G*.
> Daniel sits on the *table*.
> The *nurse listens* to Daniel.
> The *nurse* does a *poke*.
> Daniel goes home.

When they arrive at the office, Nana gives the nurse a short note to give to Dr. Gerard before they meet her. It has a photo of Daniel and reads:

> Hi! My name is Daniel, and my favorite things are basketball and my stuffed giraffe, Lolly. I have moderate cognitive impairment. Sometimes I'm really hyper and don't pay attention as well as other kids. Although I'm four years old, I do things more like a two- or three-year-old. I don't understand long descriptions. Please use short words and sentences for me. I can understand two-step directions. I call you Dr. G. I call a stethoscope a "listen" and shots "pokes." If you get too close, sometimes I might hit you. Nana can help explain things to me and help me in my appointment if you explain to her what you need to do.

Dr. G is excited to meet Daniel and very appreciative of Nana's note. She asks Daniel about basketball and his giraffe, Lolly. Dr. G is careful to use short phrases to describe to Daniel and Nana what she is doing during the exam. She says later that the note really helped her and the nurse understand how to better interact with Daniel. The appointment goes smoothly, and Daniel even hugs Dr. G at the end.

QUESTIONS TO ASK YOURSELF

- What do I think is my child's level of cognitive impairment?
- What are my child's unique strengths, weaknesses, and interests?
- How will I need to adapt the strategies to fit my child?

ACTION STEPS

- In your C.O.A.C.H. notebook, write a script like the example of the one Nana used to share with your child's medical providers.
- List the strategies you've tried, for how long, and your sense of if they've helped or not.
- Note any changes you could make to the strategies you're using or new ones to add based on your child's unique needs.

28

Children Who Are Nonverbal or Who Have Communication Needs

> Some people with autism may not be able to speak or answer to their name, but they can still hear your words and feel your kindness.
>
> —Everyday Power website

When children have difficulty communicating with the world around them, it can be challenging to meet their needs. It can be particularly tough to adapt their medical care in ways that best fit them. Some medical providers are skilled at assessing and treating children who are nonverbal; others simply haven't had the training or experience to optimize the child's (and parents') medical experiences. In these cases, it is even more important for parents to advocate for their child. Parents can help bridge the gap between their child's needs and the medical team's ability to meet these needs.

There are a number of tools that parents can use to help maximize their child's ability to communicate with their medical team. As a start, think about the tools that you may use in everyday life. How do you communicate with your child at home? What works best? What doesn't work? What increases frustration or stress in your child? What helps your child relax? Consider bringing these tools or adapting them to use with your child's medical team.

Examples of tools that may be helpful in a medical context include the integration of technology, picture cards, and visual schedules. There are a number of communication technology tools that facilitate communication by having children select letters, words, or pictures. Some children can use computers to type information or to point to choices. If your child uses one of these tools at home or in school, consider bringing it to medical appointments as well.

Visual schedules can be used to visually depict the plan for the day. You can work with your child to show them what to expect at the doctor's office so that they will be prepared. In the hospital, you may be able to work with child life specialists or nurses to create word or picture boards. This can help your child know what to expect and help them participate in their care.

If you have a child who is nonverbal or who communicates differently than expected, you may also be able to help your child communicate discomfort or pain based on observation. Think about your child: How do they express discomfort? How do you tell the difference between your child fighting something because they are in pain and fighting something because they don't want to do it? This isn't always clear, so it is okay if you don't know. Watch for body responses: increased heart rate, becoming flushed, increased sweating, or tightening muscles. Also consider emotional responses: increased irritability, increased sadness, or decreased cooperation. Consider making a list of signs that you've seen in your child that seem to be related to pain. Share these with your child's medical team.

How do you tell the difference between your child fighting something because they are in pain and fighting something because they don't want to do it?

Jin's Communication

When we first met Jin, we learned that she has communication challenges. Initially, we were not sure if Jin's communication challenges were related to a language barrier or to a developmental disability or other medical condition. Some of Jin's early fears at the doctor's office seemed to be related to her not understanding what was going on.

As Jin's speech therapist begins to work with her, she recommends that Jin's family start using visual schedules for daily routines. She also suggests that they use picture cards to allow Jin to make some choices. Jin's parents decide to also make cards with words and pictures on them to help Jin know when she has appointments. They make cards showing each step of the appointment. Jin's parents also make big YES and NO cards to use when she has a choice. These cards help Jin communicate both at home and at medical appointments.

QUESTIONS TO ASK YOURSELF

- What type of communication tools work best for my child?
- What's working with my child's communication? What's not working? Do I need to look for other ways to help my child communicate with their medical team?

ACTION STEPS

- In your C.O.A.C.H. notebook, make a list of ways that your child communicates that are unique.
- Share one communication tool with your child's doctor.
- Talk with your child's primary doctor if you need help finding communication tools specific for your child.

29

Very Young Children

> When little people are overwhelmed by big emotions, it's our job to share our calm, not join their chaos.
>
> —L. R. Knost, The Gottman Institute

Parents of infants and toddlers have the unique challenge of trying to differentiate medical trauma from developmentally appropriate behavioral challenges and other changes.[1,2] If your child is an infant or toddler, you may find it helpful to focus on the observation step in the C.O.A.C.H. process. At this age, your child's behaviors are how they express their emotional reactions.

Trauma may look different in a very young child. In addition to the signs in older children that we mentioned earlier, trauma can look like

- being more difficult to soothe,
- eating poorly or losing weight,
- unusually high levels of distress when they are separated from you,
- difficulties with social connection,
- difficulty learning, or
- physical symptoms such as stomachaches.[3]

Because young children often already have trouble detaching from their primary caregiver, and often go through different stages of development and emotions, it can be difficult to differentiate trauma from typical childhood changes.

POTENTIAL CAUSES OF BEHAVIOR CHANGES

Depending on the behaviors observed that suggest medical trauma, there are a number of possible explanations for the challenges described above. For example, separation anxiety generally occurs because the child feels unsafe in some way. Ask yourself whether this is happening in specific places, with specific people, or all the time. Has there been a situation where your child left your care and felt unsafe? Has anything recently thrown your child's world off balance, made them feel afraid, or upset their typical routine? If separation occurred in the context of medical care, that's definitely something to consider as part of medical trauma. If there are other potential stressors, it may not relate to medical care.

For physical challenges such as poor eating or even being difficult to soothe, observe whether these behaviors come and go or if they are a consistent challenge. If they persist, talk with your child's doctor. There are many potential medical causes that your doctor can help you rule out or confirm.

While it may be difficult at times to distinguish typical childhood changes, challenges caused by another source, and medical trauma, the strategies described in this book will support your child's emotional development even if the source of the challenge is not trauma. Trying one or more strategies is a great way to start. You may be able to prevent future trauma symptoms by starting early.

ADAPTING THE STRATEGIES

Key interventions for very young children dealing with medical trauma include planning ahead, distraction, and reinforcement. Everything takes extra time with young children. That is doubly true when it comes to medical care. If you end up rushing a young child, sometimes it actually takes longer. This can cause even more delay and stress for both of you. Allow extra time for very young children. Try to avoid naptime when scheduling appointments. Have a stocked "go bag" for doctor appointments and hospital trips so you don't forget needed snacks and activities. Try a visual schedule (when they are old enough) to help them understand what is going to happen.

Distraction can also look different for a young child. If you are nursing or the child takes a bottle, sometimes you can feed them during certain procedures such as shots or blood draws. Playing games like peek-a-boo or blowing and popping bubbles can work too. While screen time isn't recommended for young children, you may consider making an exception for a medical appointment. A funny video might provide enough distraction for a quick medical exam or procedure. Distraction for a young child will still require some advance planning, but you can also throw in a funny dance or a goofy face in a pinch.

Very young children thrive with positive reinforcement like eye contact, praise, and hugs. Reinforcement can be less complicated for a toddler than for an older child. They don't yet understand complex cause and effect and their memories are not fully developed, so reinforcement needs to occur right away. For example, when they sit still for a shot, immediately tell them how brave they are and give them a big hug.

Daniel's Journey

Sometime when Daniel was three, Nana started noticing that he clung to her whenever people stopped by their house. All of a sudden, he became her shadow. It was the same at the hospital. The doctor had trouble peeling him away to even listen to his heart. He hid behind her leg if she put him down and wanted her to pick him back up. Nana felt terrible when he cried and tried to hold on to her. She just wanted to help him feel better. Daniel had even taken to coming out of his room soon after she put him down for his nap, crying and looking for her.

Nana knows that separation anxiety is common in young children, but it seems to have come on suddenly. They had recently taken Daniel for his vaccinations. Nana worries that maybe it had scared him. But then she also remembers that Daniel's mother had stopped by a few weeks ago to see him. This was the first visit in a couple of months. Daniel seemed cautious about his mom, but his mom insisted on holding him and taking him outside to play. Nana cleaned up from lunch while they played. From the moment Daniel came back in, he didn't leave Nana's side until his mother left. Nana wonders if Daniel's mother stopping by so unexpectedly may have caused this recent bout of separation anxiety.

Nana decides to keep reassuring him and to continue their daily routines. She is attentive but consistent when she has to separate from him. After a few weeks, Daniel is able to more easily separate and even stops getting up from his nap.

QUESTIONS TO ASK YOURSELF

- What behavior changes am I seeing that concern me?
- Are these behaviors persisting? Have I explored possible causes other than medical trauma?
- What are some ways to distract my child for ten seconds? One minute? Five minutes?

ACTION STEPS

- In your C.O.A.C.H. notebook, list the things you need to do when preparing for your child's next medical appointment.
- Try several different reinforcement strategies with your child and see what gets the best response. Jot notes down in your notebook.

Part 6

CAN PARENTS DEVELOP MEDICAL TRAUMA TOO?

30

Medical Trauma in Parents

> Watching your child suffer the horrors of treatment [for cancer] in order to have a chance at life is something no parent should ever have to experience.
>
> —Kristin, mother of Conner, twenty months old at diagnosis with atypical teratoid rhabdoid tumor

Parents (and siblings, grandparents, and anyone closely involved in a child's care) can and often do experience medical trauma reactions. When a child has a medical condition, it affects the entire family. Many parents don't recognize their own risk for developing medical trauma as they care for their child. However, across different types of medical conditions, 30 percent of parents develop significant trauma reactions.[1] In a study of 119 mothers and 52 fathers of children with cancer, all but one reported trauma reactions.[2] Similarly, in the early aftermath of a child's injury, 80 percent of parents report at least one medical trauma symptom.[3] Similar to the trauma reaction symptoms that can occur in children, parents can develop symptoms of reexperiencing, avoidance, hyperarousal, and overall changes in their mood. (Review chapter 5 for a full description of symptoms.)[4]

When a child has a medical condition, it affects the entire family.

Reexperiencing can manifest in a number of ways. Parents may experience moments or conversations replaying over and over in their mind. The moment that they learned of their child's diagnosis is a common one for many parents. Sometimes parents get stuck thinking back and blaming themselves that they "should have done this or should have gotten medical attention sooner or maybe if they would have . . . things would be different." These types of thoughts can create more anxiety for parents and get in the way of concentration. Parents may also have dreams about their experience with their child's medical condition or about fears related to a medical challenge their child is experiencing.

Avoidance can be a very tough medical trauma reaction for parents to manage. Sometimes avoidance can result in parents missing important information from doctors or medical appointments for their child. Sometimes when parents try to avoid thinking about their child's medical condition, they might forget to give their child important medications. Avoidance can also result in missing opportunities to support your child in their medical challenges. Avoidance can also be difficult if one family member wants to talk about the medical condition and the other wants to think about it as little as possible. This can become a conflict between spouses or between co-caregivers (e.g., grandparents, two parents).

Hyperarousal symptoms can make it difficult for parents to sleep well and to stay calm in general. When your body is in a fight-flight-freeze response, you are more likely to be impatient and irritable. It also makes it difficult to stay calm during a high-anxiety procedure or challenge with your child. The exact purpose of the fight-flight-freeze response is to get your body ready to do just that: fight, run away, or freeze in place. If something stressful happens when your body is in this state, the natural response is more aggression or panic.

When you are dealing with a child's serious medical condition, your overall mood can also take a hit. Parents may become more anxious, depressed, irritable, or angry. It can be hard to manage daily challenges of life when your mood is off, much less the daily challenges of having a child who is dealing with a medical condition.

TRAUMA TRIGGERS

When people are experiencing medical trauma reactions, they often develop "triggers." Triggers are things that may cause you to experience your medical trauma reactions in the moment. Reactions could include hyperarousal and panicky feelings in your body. Reactions could bring about thoughts related to your child's medical condition and your family's journey. When you are not aware of and prepared for triggers, you can be caught off guard. Recognizing your own triggers can help you be better prepared for your reactions. With this knowledge, you can plan ways to manage your reactions.

If you can recognize your own triggers, you can plan ways to manage your reactions.

Types of trauma triggers include the following:

- **Times of year:** Different times of year may remind you of your child's diagnosis or a particularly challenging part of their illness or treatment.
- **Holidays and birthdays:** Holidays are often a time of reflection. For many people, the holidays can be reminders of how things might have changed since their child's diagnosis, injury, or other medical challenge. Holidays can also bring on thoughts of how we wish things were different. Even positive events, such as graduations or weddings, can bring out strong emotions for parents as you remember the journey that you have walked with your child.
- **Places:** Any place that your mind associates with a particularly difficult part of your child's medical condition can become a trigger. This could include rooms in your home, doctors' offices, hospital rooms, the hospital itself, the exit of the highway, or anywhere else that holds meaning for you.
- **People:** Some people may remind you of the challenges of your child's health. These people could be either positive or negative and still be triggers. For example, a friend that showed up for you when you were falling apart is positive but could remind you of the tough time. A medical provider who you didn't care for could trigger you. A doctor who saved your child's life could trigger you even though they played a positive role.
- **Smells:** Have you ever noticed how smells can quickly take you back to a memory? For example, smelling a particular cookie baking might bring you back to childhood holiday memories. The same is true for traumatic memories. Sometimes certain medications, cleaners, or places have a smell that gets encoded into your mind and takes you back to that place with a single whiff.

- **Sounds:** Sounds are also common trauma triggers. Like the other triggers, anything that your mind associates with a trauma can be a trigger. For example, some parents might become hyperaware if they hear a child cough, hospital machines beeping, ambulance sirens, or Life Flight helicopters. There might be a song or a movie from the time of their life when their child was diagnosed that brings them back to those emotions.

If you can recognize your own triggers, you can plan what to do when you are faced with a trigger. Planning ahead can empower you to better manage your medical trauma reactions.

How do you know if you need more help with your medical trauma reactions? Some hints:

- Your reactions are difficult to deal with.
- Your reactions are getting in the way of you accomplishing what you want or need to do. For example, you are having trouble parenting the way you want, working, taking care of your home, or getting along with a partner.
- Others are telling you they are worried about you.

Take a look at the checklist later in this chapter for a brief self-assessment.

There are some very good evidence-based treatments that can help you overcome trauma symptoms. Some of these treatments include trauma-focused cognitive behavioral therapy, cognitive processing therapy, and prolonged exposure therapy.[5]

Maria (Nia's Mother)

Nia's mother, Maria, has been struggling through Nia's illness. From the moment Nia was diagnosed, Maria's whole world turned upside down. Maria lived her entire life for her girls. The thought of possibly losing Nia was devastating. Maria was bothered by every treatment, every fight, and every moment of managing Nia's illness.

But, as always, Maria tries to put her own feelings away and focus on supporting her girls. She avoids questions about how Nia is doing, usually trying to change the subject. She tries not to think about it at all. Sometimes she has dreams about when the doctor told her, "Nia has cancer." Maria sometimes doesn't sleep well and has trouble focusing at work. She often jumps when her phone rings, worried that it is the doctor with more bad news. She knows she needs to talk to the doctors, but sometimes she avoids them. It can be too much to carry. She feels crazy with her thoughts constantly running through her head. Missing sleep only makes it worse.

Maria first started to learn about medical trauma reactions through her girls. As she starts to help them, she wonders if she is the only parent who feels this way. One afternoon, one of her daughter's favorite nurses sits down with her and asks her how she is doing. In that moment, all the feelings that she had been trying to keep away to be brave for her daughter come rushing out. Maria starts crying and admits that she has been struggling. The nurse helps her understand that this happens to many parents. She is not alone. She is not the only one. The nurse mentions to Maria that some parents go to support groups or to therapy to get help as a parent of a child with cancer. Just knowing she is not alone and not crazy is Maria's first step in starting to recognize and deal with her own medical trauma reactions. Maria is forever grateful to this nurse.

QUESTIONS TO ASK YOURSELF

- Am I experiencing medical trauma reactions?
- Do I have any trauma triggers? What happens in my body and mind when I am triggered?

ACTION STEPS

- Determine whether you have medical trauma reactions. Go through the medical trauma checklist on the next page to help you figure it out.
- In your C.O.A.C.H. notebook, create a section for yourself. Write down trauma symptoms if you have any. Make a list of your trauma triggers.
- If you need help, ask your doctor for ideas or a referral.

CAREGIVER MEDICAL TRAUMA CHECKLIST

This checklist provides a list of possible symptoms of medical trauma that caregivers may experience. It is not a replacement for being evaluated by a professional. If you experience any of the symptoms below, this could be a sign of medical trauma. Talk with your doctor if you are concerned about these symptoms or if these symptoms are getting in the way of you doing what you need to or want to do. Ask your doctor to help with a referral to a counselor or discuss other treatment options.

_____ I think about my child's medical condition or medical care almost all the time.
_____ I try to refuse to talk about my child's condition or medical care.
_____ I get upset when talking about my child's condition or medical care.
_____ I have dreams about my child's medical condition or experiences my family has had with my child's medical care.
_____ I have frequent nightmares about my child's medical condition or treatments.
_____ My body has strong reactions (such as racing heart, fast breathing, stomachache) when I am reminded of my child's medical condition.
_____ I feel mad a lot.
_____ I feel bad a lot.
_____ I feel sad a lot.
_____ I worry a lot.
_____ I am really jumpy.
_____ I have trouble sleeping.
_____ I have trouble concentrating.
_____ I make us late to medical appointments.
_____ I avoid talking to my child's medical team whenever possible.

31

What's "Wrong" with Me?

> Sometimes when I say "I'm okay," I want someone to look me in the eyes, hug me tight, and say, "I know you are not."
>
> —Unknown

After going through the checklist at the end of the last chapter, maybe you've recognized that you are experiencing some symptoms of medical trauma. Maybe there are times when you just want to fall apart, but you can't because you are the one holding it all together for your child and family.

You are not alone. We see you. You and your child are why we wrote this book.

We want to share some other situations that parents have experienced so you can see that you are not alone. We're going to revisit our four families to dive deeper into situations of reexperiencing, avoidance, hyperarousal, and changes in overall mood.

REEXPERIENCING—DANIEL'S MOM

Sandy remembers everything about the room where the doctor told her that her son was sick and probably going to die. The drab yellow paint on the walls had begun to peel down by the corner baseboard.

Daniel is sleeping blissfully on her lap but suddenly feels heavy. It is like the weight of the doctor's words is suddenly leaning against her chest. Her breathing becomes shallow. She just wants to curl up into herself and pretend this isn't happening. She stares at Daniel's little face. She can't make sense of the fact that the doctor is saying he has this terrible disease and that he will probably die before he is fifteen years old.

"Are you okay? Do you need me to call someone?" The doctor tilts his head to the side, concerned. Sandy shakes her head slowly. She grabs the papers he holds out to her. The lady sitting next to her, a genetic counselor, touches her shoulder and offers a knowing look. She has white hair, a kind face, and sad eyes, as if she too had been in a room like this once upon a time.

You are not alone.

Sandy is supposed to bring Daniel back to her parents' house after the appointment so she can head back to work. Instead she drives back home in a daze. She heats up some dinner for Daniel. She texts her mom to tell her that she isn't feeling well. After dinner, she puts Daniel to sleep in the crib next to her bed, lies down, and drifts off.

She wakes up thinking that she just had a nightmare. She looks over at Daniel, and he is perfect. His lips are just starting to move in that pre-cry she knows so well. She is so lucky to have such a perfect child.

Bam! The realization slams into her like an eighteen-wheeler going ninety miles an hour. Her chest clenches, and all of a sudden she remembers. "No, no, no, no." She gulps as the sobs rack her body. He isn't perfect after all. He is sick. Very, very sick. She rolls back onto the bed just as Daniel lets out a loud wail.

AVOIDANCE—CAMERON'S DAD

Sitting in the waiting room during Cameron's first surgery to set the bones in his legs, Cameron's dad, Preston, focuses on his laptop. He props his cell phone on his shoulder. Zoe is annoyed that Preston can't just sit there with her and talk while Cameron is in such an important surgery. But Preston works, and she flips through a waiting-room magazine again and again.

When they are finally called in to see Cameron in recovery, Preston suggests that Zoe go back first since she is better at comforting

Cameron. Truth be told, Preston doesn't want to see Cameron with tubes and wires coming out of him. This has to get better, he thinks. It will surely just be a few weeks until life goes back to normal.

Zoe is back with Cameron for some time. When she finally comes out, she tells Preston that they are transferring Cameron to a hospital room. She says he'll probably be in the hospital for at least another week or two. Preston volunteers to run home and get the things that Zoe and Cameron will need for the hospital stay. He *doesn't do* hospitals, so they both know Zoe will be staying.

Over the next week, Preston occasionally stops by after work for a few minutes. If he is awake, Cameron is usually watching TV or playing a game on his iPad. Preston reasons that he doesn't need to be there long. He isn't sure what the plan is for after the hospital, but he is afraid it will be challenging. He doesn't even want to ask. One night when Preston stops by after work, Zoe tells him that Cameron will still be in a wheelchair when he is discharged. Then Cameron will start intensive rehab. Preston just nods his head. He can't even think about it. What if his son never walks again?

HYPERAROUSAL—JIN'S MOM

After that first visit to the emergency room and Jin's diagnosis with diabetes, Amy worries almost every day. When Jin starts school, Amy fears that Jin will have a problem with her blood sugar at school. Every time her phone rings, Amy worries that it will be the school nurse saying that Jin's blood sugar is out of control and she's called an ambulance. Weeks go by and the call never comes, but Amy still holds her breath every time she answers the phone.

Amy often feels like she is waiting for the other shoe to drop.

On the weekends, Amy has become obsessive about checking Jin's blood sugar. When Jin is tired, Amy is afraid that her blood sugar is low and she might be ready to go into diabetic shock. When Jin eats a lot of carbs in one meal, Amy furiously calculates the insulin adjustment required. Amy sometimes scolds Jin for not taking her diabetes seriously. Afterward, Amy sometimes goes into her room and cries, not knowing why she is blaming Jin. It is all so overwhelming.

When Jin's teacher calls to suggest that Jin get evaluated for speech therapy at school, Amy practically jumps down her throat.

She tells the teacher that they are already taking care of that in private therapy. Amy doesn't know why she became so defensive. This teacher has been great with Jin. She knows the teacher is only trying to help her daughter.

Amy is on edge. A lot.

OVERALL MOOD CHANGES—NIA'S MOM

Maria peeks through the glass in the door to see what this support group really looks like. She doesn't want to spend the evening in a pity party with fifteen other parents. Is she going to be the only single mother? What if some of the kids are doing really badly? She isn't sure if this is the place for her, but she forces herself to check it out.

Maria sits in her chair with her head down at first, listening to some of the other stories. Her mind keeps coming back to her own daughter, comparing their situations to hers. Is her daughter doing better or worse? Is her cancer more treatable or less? Are they on the same medications?

Finally, it's her turn. As she starts to describe the journey they've been on since Nia's diagnosis, it all comes out like a flood. Pretty soon, someone is passing the box of tissues as Maria talks about just how sad she is. She is sad for Nia, and she is sad for herself. She is sad for her daughter Sara. She misses the life they were supposed to be living.

Maria's friends at work have started to notice that she has stopped going out to lunch with them. They'll try to crack a joke, and she just stares back. Things aren't very funny anymore. What has happened to the old Maria, she wonders.

YOUR FAMILY

Does your story sound like any of these? Again, you are not alone in feeling this way. Each of these caregivers has struggled with symptoms of medical trauma and has had a hard time putting their finger on exactly what is wrong. The good news is that, once you recognize it, you can do something about it.

QUESTIONS TO ASK YOURSELF

- How am I doing with all this?
- How are others in my family handling everything?

ACTION STEPS

- In your C.O.A.C.H. notebook or in a separate journal, make some notes about anything that you are currently struggling with.
- Continue reading to learn more strategies for managing emotional reactions to your child's medical condition.

32

How Can I Support Myself?

> Showing your children that you matter, you have worth and are entitled to self-love, is one of the best ways to teach your kids how to value themselves.
>
> —Renee Brown

Oh good! You are reading this chapter! To be honest, it is debatable whether this chapter should be at the very end where it is or if it should be the very first chapter. Taking care of yourself is the most important thing you can do. It helps you care for your child. You know when you are on an airplane and the flight attendant explains how to put on oxygen masks in case of an emergency? You are supposed to put yours on first before helping others. If you don't and you pass out, then there's no one left to help. The same concept applies to parenting . . . especially a child with a medical condition. If parents do not take care of themselves, everyone suffers, including their child.

Even as we type this, we can hear many of you saying, "There's no time," "It's not possible," "My child's needs are more important," "I don't have any energy left for myself." We know these responses because (1) we are parents and (2) we have met thousands of parents of children with medical challenges.

But humor us for just a quick thousand words.

When we talk about taking care of yourself so that you can best care for your child, we don't mean that you need to put yourself ahead of all others. We don't mean you need to claim hours and hours of "me time." We mean do what you can. Do what you need to. Think carefully about what works best for you to help you feel good or better. If you don't try, there is a 100 percent guarantee that it won't happen.

SELF-CARE JUMP-START

Here are a few steps you can take to get started:

Step 1: Think about your needs. Estimated time needed: five to ten minutes.

Often, as parents of children with medical challenges, we forget or feel unable to take the time to even think about what we need. Think about different parts of your life. Can you take your coffee outside for five minutes? Can you take a minute to think while you are getting food ready for your child?

What do you need physically? What do you need emotionally? Spiritually? Financially? Socially?

Five minutes not long enough? Keep going or find another five minutes later.

Step 2: Pay attention to yourself.

Do what you can. Do what you need to.

What are the signs and signals that you are feeling stress? Do you have trouble sleeping? Do you sleep more? Do you get snappy or agitated? Do you withdraw? Do you eat more? Do you eat less?

Recognizing when you need to take action is key. If you can figure out your own signs, then you can figure out when you need to do something to prevent or deal with stress.

Step 3: Brainstorm self-care ideas. Estimated time needed: at least thirty seconds.

What can you do in thirty seconds? In two minutes? In thirty minutes? If you had a whole day? A weekend?

Can you take five deep breaths? Find an uplifting quote of the day or joke of the day app? Go to the bathroom alone? Take a shower? Call a friend? Take a walk? Watch a ball game? Do yoga in your child's hospital room? Write in a journal? Go for a hike? Do something with your child that *you* love?

The key is to do what *you* need, not what you think you should be doing. Not what others find helpful. Yoga and meditation stresses some people out, while others live by it. Figure out what works for *you* and make it a priority. Try to do something small for yourself every day.

Step 4: Start

Just start. It can be thirty seconds of a crossword puzzle, meditation, calling a friend, or watching a sports event. If it gets interrupted, try again later.

BARRIERS TO SELF-CARE

By now, your brain may be rattling off all the reasons why it's a challenge to care for yourself. Although many of those reasons may sound valid, try to fight against using them to dismiss this process. Many of us have spent years caring for all those around us while not taking care of ourselves.

Maybe these common reasons that parents struggle with self-care are in your head:

I don't have time! This is a very common response. And we really don't have time; we have to make time. We might be overloaded with demands from doctors, insurance companies, therapists, and just the day-to-day parenting responsibilities. Making ourselves a priority is one way to both care for our child and not lose our identity in the process. Remember how part 2 of this book talked about the various roles you play? The first and core role is *you* as a person. Start small with just a few minutes a day or thirty minutes once a week to care for yourself.

It feels selfish! This is a thought that might run through our minds (or unfortunately, friends or family might tell us this). If you want to blame this book for insisting that you take care of yourself, do it. Taking care of yourself—physically, mentally, emotionally, and spiritually—is not selfish. Say this ten times: "Self-care is not selfish." If you aren't able to grab on to it for yourself, grab on to it for your child.

Think back to one of the tough moments with your child. Maybe they were fighting against getting a needlestick. Maybe they were running away from you in the grocery store. Maybe they were having a full-blown meltdown in the middle of a family party. When you go into these situations completely drained, you are more likely to be less patient and have a harder time. If you have some energy left or have taken some time for yourself, you may be able to approach these challenges with a bit more understanding, patience, and grace.

What do you need every day to feel calmer and centered? Figuring that out is your first step. Then work it into your life. If you break down, the system breaks down.

While there will likely be moments when you need to put everything else aside to care for your child or to support them through a medical procedure, try to also care for yourself. *Keep at least one thing that you enjoy going in your life.*

Nia's Mom—Taking Time for Self-Care

If you've read Nia's family's story throughout the book, you may guess that Maria is very focused on supporting her children. In addition, as a single full-time working mother, her plate is quite full trying to manage everything day in and day out. Maria often neglects to take care of herself throughout Nia's battle with cancer. In truth, she wasn't really taking care of herself well even before Nia became ill.

As Maria begins to develop medical trauma symptoms and understand the long journey that Nia's cancer battle will require, she starts to feel like she is falling apart. She feels like she really needs to get more sleep and get help with caring for her children. But it just isn't possible in her situation.

After getting really frustrated with a nurse one afternoon, Maria realizes that her current approach isn't working. She thought she was doing the right thing by racing straight from work to the hospital. However, this is creating too much stress. She isn't making time to eat. She never slows down.

So while Nia is in the hospital, Maria decides to pack her dinner. She starts spending twenty minutes sitting in her car in the parking lot by herself. She listens to music and eats her dinner. Then she picks up Sara and heads to the hospital to stay with Nia. By the time she picks up Sara, she is feeling calmer, which helps Sara as well. Maria finds that taking twenty minutes to herself improves her mood, helps her be more patient, and allows her to better enjoy time with her daughters.

Daniel's Grandparents—Different Needs

Daniel's grandparents prioritize Daniel above all else. They feel guilty that his mother has left him in their care. They are doing everything they can to show him love and support. One of the biggest struggles for both of them is fatigue. Nana is retired and takes care of Daniel full time. Papa had retired but recently took a new job to help cover medical expenses for Daniel. During Daniel's intensive medical phases, they both end up exhausted. Sometimes they take this out on each other, becoming snappy and irritable.

During one appointment, Nana notices someone knitting in the waiting room. She had knitted in the past but hadn't found time in recent years. Seeing another caregiver knitting reminds her of how calming she used to find it. She decides to pick it back up to have something productive to do during many of Daniel's appointments. She decides to knit hats and baby blankets and donate them to the children's hospital. While this does not help with her tiredness, it does bring her calmness. She feels good about giving to others as well.

Papa knows that what he needs is some time alone. Between working and trying to help with Daniel, weeks often go by where he is never alone. After an evening recently in which he blew up and started yelling at everyone, he realizes he needs something to be different. Working with Nana, they figure out a way for him to have thirty minutes to himself each night after he returns home from work. Papa finds that this thirty minutes makes a huge difference in his ability to manage the multiple stresses of work and helping to care for Daniel.

QUESTIONS TO ASK YOURSELF

- What are my current biggest stressors?
- What do I notice in myself when I start to become stressed?
- What types of things bring me feelings of calm or peace?

ACTION STEPS

- In your C.O.A.C.H. notebook, brainstorm self-care ideas.
- Choose one idea and start it today or this coming weekend.

Part 7

WRAPPING UP

33

Seeking More Help

> There's no point in being complete on the outside when you're broken on the inside.
>
> —Nick Vujicic

You've almost reached the end of this book! We hope you've learned quite a bit about strategies to support your child, your family, and yourself.

This book has shared with you the tools to help prevent or reduce medical trauma in your child and even in yourself, but sometimes we all have greater needs. Where do we go if we've tried lots of strategies from this book and we're still struggling? Or where might we go alongside working these strategies?

Remember that this book is not a replacement for professional help. Take a look at the resources mentioned below. If you need more help, ask your child's medical team or your own doctor.

FOR YOUR CHILD

We've mentioned several potential resources for your child throughout this book, but let's review them here.

Child Life Services

If your hospital or clinic has child life specialists, these medical team members are often the frontline workers in helping your child with medical trauma issues. They are trained in child development and strategies to support your child through some medical challenges. Using play and education, they can partner with you, provide tangible resources during appointments or hospital stays, and support you and your child through education. They can also act as a liaison with the medical team in explaining your child's unique needs.

Social Workers

Some doctors' offices and hospitals have social workers who are trained in counseling to help support your child and family through the challenges of a medical journey. Others have social workers who are experts in finding helpful resources for families—anything from referrals for more help to parking vouchers to help with insurance challenges and beyond.

Hospital or Clinic-Based Psychologists

Some children's hospitals and medical centers have psychologists with training or expertise in pediatric medical trauma on staff. They are often called pediatric psychologists. They may be available when your child is in the inpatient hospital, for outpatient needs, or both. Pediatric psychologists evaluate your child's emotional reactions to their medical condition. They can help you sort out if preexisting or other new mental health conditions need to be addressed in your child. Many of them are trained in medical trauma symptoms and can create a specialized plan for your child, possibly incorporating many of the strategies we've discussed here. Depending on your medical setting, they also may be able to offer ongoing therapy for your child.

Pediatric psychologists evaluate your child's emotional reactions to their medical condition.

There are also neuropsychologists who can evaluate your child's cognitive and executive functioning. For some medical conditions, evaluations before or early in treatment and after treatment are built into care. For other conditions, you may need to request an evaluation.

Community Therapists

Your local community may also have therapists specifically equipped to deal with types of trauma. If you are looking for a therapist in the community, consider checking with your insurance company for a list of covered providers. Then consider finding someone who works regularly with kids the age of your child. If your child is having trauma symptoms, consider a therapist who offers cognitive behavioral therapy, trauma-focused cognitive behavioral therapy, or parent-child interaction therapy. Other supportive therapies could include talk therapy, play therapy, art therapy, or music therapy. If you can find a therapist who has worked with children with medical conditions, that can be helpful. If not, you can offer to provide them information on your child's medical condition or challenges.

Medications

There may be an occasion where your child's physician or therapist might recommend one or more medications to help with your child's anxiety or other trauma-based symptoms. Medication used in addition to other strategies (such as those recommended in this book) can make things easier for some children. Ask questions to understand the goals of the medication, dosing, and whether the doctor expects it to be ongoing or for a short period.

Support Groups

There may be support groups in your area or online for children with high medical needs or children with your child's specific condition. Sometimes even a more general support group at a local therapy practice may be an option for some children. Start by asking at your local hospital or therapy practice, searching online, or asking other parents who are facing similar challenges. Some may be active, whereas others may offer periodic group experiences where children can process as they enjoy activities and build relationships.

Sibling Support Groups

Some hospitals or disease communities offer support groups or experiences for siblings of children with unique health challenges.

Ask your hospital's child life services team about it, or you can search online using the key term "sibling support" and your affected child's condition or your local major health care institution.

Online Resources

There are many reputable online resources. For example, the National Child Traumatic Stress Network and the International Society for Traumatic Stress Studies offer online resources that might be helpful in addition to those discussed in this book. The Center for Pediatric Traumatic Stress also offers resources through HealthCareToolBox.org. Ask your medical team for more resources specific to your child's medical condition.

FOR YOU

Some of the same resources listed above for your child, such as hospital-based psychologists and support groups, may also focus on you as an individual as well as part of the family. Below are several additional options for you to specifically address medical trauma issues.

If you need more help, ask your child's medical team or your own doctor.

Therapists

A personal therapist who is knowledgeable in or specializes in trauma can play a valuable role in helping you process medical trauma. There are also specific evidence-based techniques, such as EMDR (eye movement desensitization and reprocessing), cognitive behavioral therapy, trauma-focused cognitive behavioral therapy, and narrative therapy, that are effective in helping with different kinds of trauma.

Support Groups

There may be support groups in your area or online for parenting in general, parenting children with special medical needs, caregiving related to your child's specific condition or group of conditions (such as childhood cancer), or trauma generally. Start by asking at your local hospital, searching online, or asking other parents who are facing similar challenges.

Online Resources

The organizations mentioned above for your child also feature online resources for parents.

Sometimes it can be difficult to reach out and ask for help. It takes strength to recognize when you are struggling and seek help to get through it. Our hope is that with the information we've provided in this book, you can recognize when you or your child need help. We encourage you to ask your medical team for more support if you need it. With the strategies in this book and the support of your medical team and others in your life, we hope you can prevent, reduce, and manage the medical trauma in your child's life and in your own. In doing this, we are rooting for your family's physical, emotional, and mental health.

34

Epilogue

Now you know the rest of the story.

—Paul Harvey

The family stories featured in this book involve characters that we have grown to love. Their stories are inspired by experiences of individuals and families we've encountered, but each of these stories is unique. If you're like us, you want to know what happens with these families. Here is where we'll tell the rest of the story.

Cameron

Prior to Cameron's injuries from the car crash, he had been a typical teenager with a very close family. His family members got along with each other most of the time and ran from school and work to extracurriculars and back again. We walked through much of Cameron's journey as he began his recovery from his injuries in the first week to the first few months. The accident, his injuries, and his recovery took a toll on his entire family. His parents worked hard to get everyone back on track and asked for help when they needed it.

Now, six months later, things are a bit more routine, and everyone is starting to live life again. Cameron still has quite a few medical appointments, including ongoing physical therapy, but he has started walking, which has really helped him to feel more optimistic. He's not back on the soccer field yet, but he can now see this as a possibility in the future. Cameron is now getting along better with his brother, Emerson, and is able to regularly enjoy his friends. Sometimes he still has some medical trauma reactions, which are most often triggered by hospital visits, but now he knows what these reactions are and how to deal with them better. Cameron also knows that his parents stood by him throughout everything and that he can reach out for help if he starts having a hard time again.

Cameron's parents, Zoe and Preston, are still working through some of their own emotional reactions to everything that happened. They have been able to come together more and work through things together. In addition, Zoe has set some time aside every week to get together with some good friends so that she can get additional social support. Preston still battles feelings of guilt, especially during soccer season, but is doing better over time. As a family, they still have growing to do, but they have been able to get to a much better place.

Nia

We met Nia; her sister, Sara; and her mother, Maria, as they were all struggling through Nia's cancer treatment. Throughout the book, we got to watch all three of them gain comfort and confidence with Nia's treatment.

At this time, Nia has entered remission and completed this round of cancer treatment. She is now back in school full time and thriving. While she still doesn't like when she has to get checked out by the doctor (especially if needles are involved), she makes it through appointments with her mother's support. She is now taking dance classes twice a week and laughing with her friends.

Sara feels better now that Nia's treatment is complete. She worries sometimes that the cancer will come back. Now, instead of hiding her fears, she talks to her mother and her school counselor. They work together to help her figure out how to deal with her worries when they pop up. Sara has also discovered that she loves to write and has started to write a book about what it was like for her to go through Nia's cancer treatment.

Maria has found that the experience of walking her child through a life-threatening illness has been life-changing for her. She has permanent worries about both of her girls, as most mothers do. She does sometimes flash back to when she first learned of Nia's cancer and remembers how terrified she was. She will always have some worries about the cancer coming back, but these worries don't control her. Now she is much less afraid of the "little stuff." During Nia's treatment, she learned how to stand up for her daughter in a whole new way. Now, if she has questions for teachers or questions at her job, she doesn't hesitate to ask. She figures, if she can get through her child's cancer, she can get through anything.

The three of them continue to carve out time to spend together and do not take the time for granted. Knowing that they could have lost Nia, they treasure their dance parties and family game nights.

Daniel

Daniel is enjoying preschool, which he attends three days each week in a classroom with children with special needs as well as typical peers. The teacher often encourages the children to share about other situations in their lives. Daniel's grandparents think that this might be a great opportunity to incorporate his medical needs with school and with his friends.

Nana and Papa use medical play to help Daniel with his weekly infusions, so he has lots of medical supplies and a favorite teddy bear that is always his patient. They practice with Daniel, and he starts getting excited that he will get to show his friends that "he is a doctor!" as Daniel says.

Nana and Papa have been updating their daughter Sandy about Daniel's progress with his treatments. Although the diagnosis and Daniel's initial medical needs had been incredibly overwhelming to Sandy, she has started reading more about Hunter syndrome lately and wants to spend more time with Daniel.

Recently, Sandy met them at the hospital for Daniel's infusion, and she and Nana talked more about what it could look like for Sandy to become more involved in Daniel's life again. Although Sandy's job makes it difficult to care for all of Daniel's needs on her own, just the fact that Sandy is now processing the grief associated with Daniel's diagnosis is a huge stride in their relationship.

When the day comes for Daniel to share with his class, Nana and Papa pick up Sandy, and they all ride together to the school. Daniel carries in his teddy bear and play doctor bag, and Sandy helps him set up in the front of the room. Although Daniel is a busy kid, buzzing around the whole time, Sandy seems to take it in stride. They work as a team—Daniel the "doctor" and Sandy the "nurse"—and show his class how Daniel gets his infusion each week at the hospital. Nana and Papa are beaming and take lots of pictures. Daniel is so proud of himself.

Nana and Papa know the journey will continue for Daniel, with new challenges as his disease progresses. The work they have done with Daniel over the past year has given them confidence that they can continue to walk with him on his path.

Jin

Now six years old, Jin is excited to enter first grade at a new school. Her language is becoming more understandable, and after touring the school, she is talking about it every day.

Her mother, Amy, scheduled a time for them to meet with the school nurse in order to walk through Jin's needs related to her diabetes. They show up with a copy of Jin's visual schedule for the nurse to use along with some special stickers and rubber bracelets to use as rewards just in case. Although Jin is shy at first, the nurse quickly draws her out of her shell with stories about school and all the fun supplies she has there at the clinic.

Amy shares with the nurse some of Jin's specific words she uses for her diabetic supplies and also brings a set of Jin's picture cards that relate to her blood sugar testing and medication. Amy likes that she and the nurse, along with Jin, are building a trusted relationship, and she feels like the nurse understands her goals for Jin's health at school. It really helps both Jin and Amy to get to know the nurse before school starts this year. Jin's parents are excited and relieved for her to be able to start school, especially now that they have been able to get the nurse's help with communication and to stabilize Jin's blood sugars.

A FINAL WRAP-UP

Thank you for honoring us by reading this book. Our hope is that by using the strategies in this book and the insights you've developed, you can continue to gain knowledge and confidence in supporting your child's care. The C.O.A.C.H. process is one that can be implemented at any time throughout your child's and your family's journey. While we are sure you will have ups and downs and maybe get turned around, we want you to know that you are not alone on your journey. Many parents have walked similar paths before you and will after you. Take it one day at a time. You can do this!

Additional Resources

If you'd like to learn more about medical trauma and how to support your child, we recommend the following resources.

BOOKS

Hall, Michelle Flaum, and Scott E. Hall. *Managing the Psychological Impact of Medical Trauma*. New York: Springer, 2016.

Scaer, Robert. *The Trauma Spectrum: Hidden Wounds and Human Resiliency*. New York: W. W. Norton, 2005.

Van der Kolk, Bessel. *The Body Keeps the Score*. New York: Penguin, 2015.

SELECTED RESEARCH ARTICLES

Doupnik, Stephanie K., Douglas Hill, Deepak Palakshappa, Diana Worsley, Hanah Bae, Aleesha Shaik, Maylene Kefeng Qiu, Meghan Marsac, and Chris Fuedtner. "Parent Coping Support Interventions during Acute Pediatric Hospitalizations: A Meta-Analysis." *Pediatrics* 140, no. 3 (2017). https://doi.org/10.1542/peds.2016-4171.

Hildenbrand, Aimee K., Scottie B. Day, and Meghan L. Marsac. "Attending to the Not-So-Little 'Little Things': Practicing Trauma-Informed Pediatric

Healthcare." *Global Pediatric Health* 6 (2019): 2333794X19879353. https://doi.org/10.1177%2F2333794X19879353.

Lerwick, Julie L. "Minimizing Pediatric Healthcare-Induced Anxiety and Trauma." *World Journal of Clinical Pediatrics* 5 (2016): 143–50. https://doi.org/10.5409/wjcp.v5.i2.143.

Marsac, Meghan L., Christine Kindler, Danielle Weiss, and Lindsay Ragsdale. "Let's Talk about It: Supporting Family Communication during End-of-Life Care of Pediatric Patients." *Journal of Palliative Medicine* 21, no. 6 (2018): 862–78. https://doi.org/10.1089/jpm.2017.0307.

Price, Julia, Nancy Kassam-Adams, Melissa A. Alderfer, Jennifer Christofferson, and Anne E. Kazak. "Systematic Review: A Reevaluation and Update of the Integrative (Trajectory) Model of Pediatric Medical Traumatic Stress." *Journal of Pediatric Psychology* 41 (2016): 86–97. https://doi.org/10.1093/jpepsy/jsv074.

ONLINE RESOURCES

After the Injury: www.aftertheinjury.org
Health Care Tool Box: www.healthcaretoolbox.org
The National Child Traumatic Stress Network: www.nctsn.org

PRODUCTS

Cellie Coping Company: www.celliecopingcompany.org

Notes

CHAPTER 1. WHERE LOVE MEETS MEDICINE

1. *Oxford English Dictionary/Lexico*, s.v. "Caring," accessed September 23, 2020, https://www.lexico.com/en/definition/caring. The origin of the word *care* is actually from the old high German form *chara*, which means grief or lament. Often our English use of the word *caring* brings about positive feelings, but at its core, our care comes from a place of identifying with our child's pain and challenges—in other words, empathy—and is the source of our desire to help.

2. Pew Research Center, "Parenting in America: Outlook, Worries, Aspirations Are Strongly Linked to Financial Situation," December 17, 2015, https://www.pewsocialtrends.org/wp-content/uploads/sites/3/2015/12/2015-12-17_parenting-in-america_FINAL.pdf.

3. Christina D. Bethell et al., "A National and State Profile of Leading Health Problems and Health Care Quality for US Children: Key Insurance Disparities and Across-State Variations," *Academic Pediatrics* 11, suppl. 3 (2011): S22–33, https://doi.org/10.1016/j.acap.2010.08.011.

4. Hatice S. Zahran et al., "Vital Signs: Asthma in Children—United States, 2001–2016," *Morbidity and Mortality Weekly Report* 67 (2018): 149–55, http://dx.doi.org/10.15585/mmwr.mm6705e1.

5. National Organization for Rare Disorders, home page, accessed September 25, 2020, https://rarediseases.org/get-involved/donate-now/give/35-years-growing/.

6. American Childhood Cancer Organization, "US Childhood Cancer Statistics," accessed September 25, 2020, https://www.acco.org/us-childhood-cancer-statistics/.

7. Centers for Disease Control and Prevention, National Center for Injury Prevention and Control, "Injury Prevention & Control: WISQARS™ Injury Data," accessed September 25, 2020, https://www.cdc.gov/injury/wisqars/index.html.

8. Andrew J. Barnes, Marla E. Eisenberg, and Michael D. Resnick, "Suicide and Self-Injury among Children and Youth with Chronic Health Conditions," *Pediatrics* 125, no. 5 (2010): 889–95, https://doi.org/10.1542/peds.2009-1814.

9. James A. Blackman et al., "Emotional, Developmental, and Behavioural Comorbidities of Children with Chronic Health Conditions," *Journal of Paediatrics and Child Health* 47, no. 10 (2011): 742–47, https://doi.org/10.1111/j.1440-1754.2011.02044.x.

10. Parminder Raina et al., "The Health and Well-Being of Caregivers of Children with Cerebral Palsy," *Pediatrics* 115, no. 6 (2015): 626–36, https://doi.org/10.1542/peds.2004-1689.

11. Naciye Vardar-Yagli et al., "Hospitalization of Children with Cystic Fibrosis Adversely Affects Mothers' Physical Activity, Sleep Quality, and Psychological Status," *Journal of Child and Family Studies* 26, no. 3 (2017): 800–9, https://doi.org/10.1007/s10826-016-0593-4.

12. Anne E. Kazak et al., "An Integrative Model of Pediatric Medical Traumatic Stress," *Journal of Pediatric Psychology* 31, no. 4 (2006): 343–55, https://doi.org/10.1093/jpepsy/jsj054.

CHAPTER 2. PARENTING THROUGH MEDICAL CHALLENGES

1. Diana Baumrind, "Effects of Authoritative Parental Control on Child Behavior," *Child Development* 37, no. 4 (1966): 887–907, https://psycnet.apa.org/doi/10.2307/1126611.

2. Eleanor E. Maccoby and John A. Martin, "Socialization in the Context of the Family: Parent-Child Interaction," in *Handbook of Child Psychology*, 4th ed., ed. Paul H. Mussen (New York: Wiley, 1983).

CHAPTER 4. WHAT EXACTLY IS MEDICAL TRAUMA?

1. Anne E. Kazak et al., "An Integrative Model of Pediatric Medical Traumatic Stress," *Journal of Pediatric Psychology* 31, no. 4 (2006): 343–55, https://doi.org/10.1093/jpepsy/jsj054.

2. American Psychiatric Association, *Diagnostic and Statistical Manual of Mental Disorders: DSM-5* (Arlington, VA: American Psychiatric Association, 2013).

3. Ulrich F. Lanius et al., eds., "Threat and Safety: The Neurobiology of Active and Passive Defense Responses," in *Neurobiology and the Treatment of Traumatic Dissociation: Toward an Embodied Self* (New York: Springer, 2014), 29–50.

4. Julia Price et al., "Systematic Review: A Reevaluation and Update of the Integrative (Trajectory) Model of Pediatric Medical Traumatic Stress," *Journal of Pediatric Psychology* 41 (2016): 86–97, https://doi.org/10.1093/jpepsy/jsv074.

5. Neil L. Schechter et al., "Pain Reduction during Pediatric Immunizations: Evidence-Based Review and Recommendations," *Pediatrics* 119 (2007): e1184–98, https://doi.org/10.1542/peds.2006-1107.

6. Christine T. Chambers et al., "Psychological Interventions for Reducing Pain and Distress during Routine Childhood Immunizations: A Systematic Review," *Clinical Therapeutics* 31, suppl. 2 (2009): s77–s103, https://doi.org/10.1016/j.clinthera.2009.07.023.

7. Anna Taddio et al., "Survey of the Prevalence of Immunization Non-Compliance Due to Needle Fears in Children and Adults," *Vaccine* 30, no. 32 (2012): 4807–12, https://doi.org/10.1016/j.vaccine.2012.05.011.

8. Mayank Kakkar et al., "Prevalence of Dental Anxiety in 10–14 Years Old Children and Its Implications," *Journal of Dental Anesthesia and Pain Medicine* 16, no. 3 (2016): 199–202, https://doi.org/10.17245/jdapm.2016.16.3.199.

9. Meghan L. Marsac et al., "The Role of Appraisals and Coping in Predicting Posttraumatic Stress Following Pediatric Injury," *Psychological Trauma: Theory, Research, Practice, and Policy* 8, no. 4 (2016): 495–503, https://dx.doi.org/10.1037/tra0000116.

10. Meghan L. Marsac et al., "Posttraumatic Stress Following Acute Medical Trauma in Children: A Proposed Model of Bio-Psycho-Social Processes during the Peri-Trauma Period," *Clinical Child and Family Psychology Review* 17, no. 4 (2014): 1–13, https://dx.doi.org/10.1007/s10567-014-0174-2.

11. Eva Alisic et al., "Building Child Trauma Theory from Longitudinal Studies: A Meta-Analysis," *Clinical Psychology Review* 31, no. 5 (2011): 736–47, https://doi.org/10.1016/j.cpr.2011.03.001.

CHAPTER 5. HOW DO I KNOW IF MY CHILD HAS MEDICAL TRAUMA?

1. Amy L. Meadows and Meghan L. Marsac, "Early Life Trauma and Diabetes Management: An Under-Recognized Phenomenon in Transition-Age

Youth," *Clinical Diabetes* 38, no. 1 (2020): 93–95, https://doi.org/10.2337/cd19-0012.

2. American Psychiatric Association, *Diagnostic and Statistical Manual of Mental Disorders: DSM-5* (Arlington, VA: American Psychiatric Association, 2013).

3. Briana Cobos, Kelly Haskard-Zolnierek, and Krista Howard, "White Coat Hypertension: Improving the Patient-Health Care Practitioner Relationship," *Psychology Research and Behavior Management* 8 (2015): 133–41, https://doi.org/10.2147/prbm.s61192.

4. Cobos et al., "White Coat Hypertension: Improving the Patient-Health Care Practitioner Relationship."

CHAPTER 6. WHAT *ISN'T* MEDICAL TRAUMA?

1. David Finkelhor, Richard Ormrod, and Heather A. Turner, "Lifetime Assessment of Poly-Victimization in a National Sample of Children and Youth," *Child Abuse and Neglect* 33, no. 7 (2009): 403–11, https://doi.org/10.1016/j.chiabu.2008.09.012.

CHAPTER 8. YOUR FAMILY AND THE HEALTH CARE SYSTEM

1. Myonghwa Park et al., "Patient- and Family-Centered Care Interventions for Improving the Quality of Health Care: A Review of Systematic Reviews," *International Journal of Nursing Studies* 87 (2018): 69–83, https://doi.org/10.1016/j.ijnurstu.2018.07.006.

2. Robert Graboyes, "Medical Paternalism in Many Guises," Mercatus Center at George Mason University, July 6, 2017, https://www.mercatus.org/essays/medical-paternalism-many-guises.

3. American Medical Association, "Code of Medical Ethics Opinion 2.2.1," accessed September 25, 2020, https://www.ama-assn.org/delivering-care/ethics/informed-consent.

4. Robert F. Graboyes and Eric Topol, *Anatomy and Atrophy of Medical Paternalism* (Arlington, VA: Mercatus Research, Mercatus Center at George Mason University, 2017), https://www.mercatus.org/system/files/mercatus-graboyes-medical-paternalism-v3_1.pdf.

CHAPTER 9. YOU ARE A PERSON, THEN A PARENT

1. Pew Research Center, "Parenting in America: Outlook, Worries, Aspirations Are Strongly Linked to Financial Situation." Decem-

ber 17, 2015, https://www.pewsocialtrends.org/wp-content/uploads/sites/3/2015/12/2015-12-17_parenting-in-america_FINAL.pdf.

2. Pew Research Center, "Parenting in America: Outlook, Worries, Aspirations Are Strongly Linked to Financial Situation."

CHAPTER 10. YOU ARE A CAREGIVER

1. Kathleen M. May, "Searching for Normalcy: Mothers' Caregiving for Low Birthweight Infants," *Pediatric Nursing* 23, no. 1 (1997): 17–20.

2. Elizabeth Kepreotes, Diana Keatinge, and Teresa Elizabeth Stone, "The Experience of Parenting Children with Chronic Health Conditions: A New Reality," *Journal of Nursing and Healthcare of Chronic Illness* 2, no. 1 (2010): 51–62, http://dx.doi.org/10.1111/j.1752-9824.2010.01047.x.

CHAPTER 11. YOU ARE THE LEADER OF YOUR CHILD'S MEDICAL TEAM

1. Elizabeth Kepreotes, Diana Keatinge, and Teresa Elizabeth Stone, "The Experience of Parenting Children with Chronic Health Conditions: A New Reality," *Journal of Nursing and Healthcare of Chronic Illness* 2, no. 1 (2010): 51–62, http://dx.doi.org/10.1111/j.1752-9824.2010.01047.x.

2. Brené Brown, "The Wholehearted Parenting Manifesto," *HuffPost*, updated November 28, 2012, https://www.huffpost.com/entry/wholehearted-parenting-manifesto_b_1923011.

CHAPTER 15. COMMUNICATION: LET'S TALK ABOUT IT

1. Meghan L. Marsac et al., "Let's Talk about It: Supporting Family Communication during End-of-Life Care of Pediatric Patients," *Journal of Palliative Medicine* 21, no. 6 (2018): 862–78, https://doi.org/10.1089/jpm.2017.0307.

2. Agathe Béranger et al., "Communication, informations et place des parents en réanimation polyvalente pédiatrique: Revue de la littérature [Communication, Information, and Roles of Parents in the Pediatric Intensive Care Unit: A Review Article]," *Archives de Pédiatrie* 24, no. 3 (2017): 265–72, https://doi.org/10.1016/j.arcped.2016.12.001.

CHAPTER 16. CONSISTENCY: KNOWING WHAT TO EXPECT

1. Susan H. Landry et al., "Does Early Responsive Parenting Have a Special Importance for Children's Development or Is Consistency across Early

Childhood Necessary?" *Developmental Psychology* 37, no. 3 (2001): 387–403, https://doi.org/10.1037/0012-1649.37.3.387.

CHAPTER 17. BEHAVIOR CHARTS: NOT BRIBING, REWARDING

1. Centers for Disease Control and Prevention, "How to Use Rewards," accessed September 25, 2020, https://www.cdc.gov/parents/essentials/consequences/rewards.html.

CHAPTER 18. ADDITIONAL VISUAL SUPPORTS: CREATIVE PREPARATION

1. Applied Behavior Analysis Programs Guide, "What Is Visual Scheduling," accessed September 25, 2020, https://www.appliedbehavioranalysisprograms.com/faq/what-is-visual-scheduling/.
2. Autism Speaks Autism Treatment Network, "Visual Supports and Autism Spectrum Disorders," accessed September 25, 2020, https://www.autismspeaks.org/sites/default/files/2018-08/Visual%20Supports%20Tool%20Kit.pdf.
3. Children's National Hospital, "Beyond the Spectrum: Visual Supports and Resources," accessed September 25, 2020, https://childrensnational.org/departments/center-for-neuroscience-and-behavioral-medicine/programs-and-services/center-for-autism-spectrum-disorders/beyond-the-spectrum/visual-supports-and-resources.

CHAPTER 20. MEDICAL PLAY: CHILDREN LEARN THROUGH PLAY

1. Kenneth R. Ginsburg, the Committee on Communications and the Committee on Psychosocial Aspects of Child and Family Health of the American Academy of Pediatrics, "The Importance of Play in Promoting Healthy Child Development and Maintaining Strong Parent-Child Bonds," *Pediatrics* 119, no. 1 (2007): 182–91, https://doi.org/10.1542/peds.2006-2697.

CHAPTER 21. ADAPTING THE ENVIRONMENT: MAKE YOURSELF AT HOME

1. Roger Ulrich et al., *The Role of the Physical Environment in the 21st Century Hospital, Report to the Center for Health Design for the Designing the 21st*

Century Hospital Project (Princeton, NJ: Robert Wood Johnson Foundation, 2004), https://www.healthdesign.org/system/files/Ulrich_Role%20of%20 Physical_2004.pdf.

2. Ulrich et al., *The Role of the Physical Environment in the 21st Century Hospital, Report to the Center for Health Design for the Designing the 21st Century Hospital Project.*

3. Chanuki Illushka Seresinhe et al., "Happiness Is Greater in More Scenic Locations," *Scientific Reports* 9 (2019): 4498, https://doi.org/10.1038/s41598-019-40854-6.

4. Rebekah Levine Coley, Alicia Doyle Lynch, and Melissa Kull, "Early Exposure to Environmental Chaos and Children's Physical and Mental Health," *Early Childhood Research Quarterly* 32, no. 3 (2015): 94–104, https://dx.doi.org/10.1016/j.ecresq.2015.03.001.

5. Ulrich et al., *The Role of the Physical Environment in the 21st Century Hospital, Report to the Center for Health Design for the Designing the 21st Century Hospital Project.*

6. Ulrich et al., *The Role of the Physical Environment in the 21st Century Hospital, Report to the Center for Health Design for the Designing the 21st Century Hospital Project.*

7. Ulrich et al., *The Role of the Physical Environment in the 21st Century Hospital, Report to the Center for Health Design for the Designing the 21st Century Hospital Project.*

8. Ulrich et al., *The Role of the Physical Environment in the 21st Century Hospital, Report to the Center for Health Design for the Designing the 21st Century Hospital Project.*

9. Kate M. Rancourt, Jill M. Chorney, and Zeev Kain, "Children's Immediate Postoperative Distress and Mothers' and Fathers' Touch Behaviors," *Journal of Pediatric Psychology* 40, no. 10 (2015): 1115–23, https://dx.doi.org/10.1093/jpepsy/jsv069.

10. Rancourt et al., "Children's Immediate Postoperative Distress and Mothers' and Fathers' Touch Behaviors."

11. Darlene A. Kertes et al., "Effect of Pet Dogs on Children's Perceived Stress and Cortisol Stress Response," *Social Development* 26, no. 2 (2017): 382–401, https://doi.org/10.1111/sode.12203.

12. Karen M. Allen et al., "Presence of Human Friends and Pet Dogs as Moderators of Autonomic Responses to Stress in Women," *Journal of Personality and Social Psychology* 61 (1991): 582–89, https://psycnet.apa.org/doi/10.1037/0022-3514.61.4.582.

CHAPTER 23. DISTRACTION: SQUIRREL!

1. Donna Koller and Ran D. Goldman, "Distraction Techniques for Children Undergoing Procedures: A Critical Review of Pediatric Research,"

Journal of Pediatric Nursing 27, no. 6 (2012): 652–81, https://doi.org/10.1016/j.pedn.2011.08.001.

2. Lindsey L. Cohen, Ronald L. Blount, and Georgia Panopoulos, "Nurse Coaching and Cartoon Distraction: An Effective and Practical Intervention to Reduce Child, Parent, and Nurse Distress during Immunizations," *Journal of Pediatric Psychology* 22, no. 3 (1997): 355–70, https://doi.org/10.1093/jpepsy/22.3.355.

3. Meghan L. Marsac et al., "An Initial Application of a Bio-Psycho-Social Framework to Predict Posttraumatic Stress Following Pediatric Injury," *Health Psychology* 36, no. 8 (2017): 787–96, https://dx.doi.org/10.1037%2Fhea0000508.

4. Alyssa C. Jones et al., "A Prospective Examination of Child Avoidance Coping and Parental Coping Assistance after Pediatric Injury: A Mixed-Methods Approach," *Journal of Pediatric Psychology* 44, no. 8 (2019): 914–23, https://doi.org/10.1093/jpepsy/jsz016.

CHAPTER 24. REINFORCEMENT: HIGH FIVE!

1. Pei-Hsuan Hsieh, "Positive Reinforcement," in *Encyclopedia of Child Behavior and Development*, ed. Sam Goldstein and Jack A. Naglieri (Boston: Springer, 2011), https://doi.org/10.1007/978-0-387-79061-9_2916.

CHAPTER 25. BODY CONTROL: MIND-BODY CONNECTION

1. Jennie C. I. Tsao et al., "Relationships among Anxious Symptomatology, Anxiety Sensitivity and Laboratory Pain Responsivity in Children," *Cognitive Behaviour Therapy* 35, no. 4 (2006): 207–15, https://doi.org/10.1080/16506070600898272.

2. Meghan L. Marsac and Jeanne B. Funk, "Relationships among Psychological Functioning, Dental Anxiety, Pain Perception, and Coping in Children and Adolescents," *Journal of Dentistry for Children* 75, no. 3 (2008): 243–51.

3. Niranga Manjuri Devanarayana et al., "Abdominal Pain–Predominant Functional Gastrointestinal Diseases in Children and Adolescents: Prevalence, Symptomatology, and Association with Emotional Stress," *Journal of Pediatric Gastroenterology and Nutrition* 53, no. 6 (2011): 659–65, https://doi.org/10.1097/mpg.0b013e3182296033.

4. National Institute of Mental Health Information Resource Center, "5 Things You Should Know about Stress," accessed September 25, 2020, https://www.nimh.nih.gov/health/publications/stress/index.shtml.

5. National Institutes of Health, National Center for Complementary and Integrative Health, "Relaxation Techniques for Health," accessed September 25, 2020, https://www.nccih.nih.gov/health/relaxation-techniques-for-health.

6. Maria Brenner et al., "Nurses' Perceptions of the Practice of Restricting a Child for a Clinical Procedure," *Qualitative Health Research* 24, no. 8 (2014): 1080–89, https://dx.doi.org/10.1177/1049732314541332.

CHAPTER 27. CHILDREN WITH COGNITIVE IMPAIRMENT

1. *A Dictionary of Psychology*, s.v. "Deviation IQ," accessed September 23, 2020, https://www.oxfordreference.com/view/10.1093/oi/authority.20110803095714395.

2. Biography.com, "What Was Albert Einstein's IQ?" accessed September 25, 2020, https://www.biography.com/news/albert-einstein-iq.

3. Lynda Lahti Anderson et al., "A Systematic Review of US Studies on the Prevalence of Intellectual or Developmental Disabilities since 2000," *Intellectual and Development Disabilities* 57, no. 5 (2019): 421–38, https://doi.org/10.1352/1934-9556-57.5.421.

4. Katherine McKenzie et al., "Systematic Review of the Prevalence and Incidence of Intellectual Disabilities: Current Trends and Issues," *Current Developmental Disorders Report* 3 (June 2016): 104–15, https://doi.org/10.1007/s40474-016-0085-7.

5. U.S. Department of Education, National Center for Education Statistics, "Table 204.30: Children 3 to 21 Years Old Served under Individuals with Disabilities Education Act (IDEA), Part B, by Type of Disability; Selected Years 1976–77 through 2017–18," *Digest of Education Statistics, 2018* (Washington, DC: National Center for Education Statistics, 2020), accessed September 25, 2020, https://nces.ed.gov/programs/digest/d18/tables/dt18_204.30.asp.

6. Committee to Evaluate the Supplemental Security Income Disability Program for Children with Mental Disorders, "Clinical Characteristics of Intellectual Disabilities," in *Mental Disorders and Disabilities among Low-Income Children*, ed. Thomas F. Boat and Joel T. Wu (Washington, DC: National Academies Press, 2015), https://www.ncbi.nlm.nih.gov/books/NBK332877/.

7. McKenzie, "Systematic Review of the Prevalence and Incidence of Intellectual Disabilities," 104.

8. Stacey Ageranioti-Bélanger et al., "Behaviour Disorders in Children with an Intellectual Disability," *Paediatrics and Child Health* 17, no. 2 (2012): 84–88, https://doi.org/10.1093/pch/17.2.84.

CHAPTER 29. VERY YOUNG CHILDREN

1. National Child Traumatic Stress Network, "How Early Childhood Trauma Is Unique," accessed September 25, 2020, https://www.nctsn.org/what-is-child-trauma/trauma-types/early-childhood-trauma/effects.

2. Substance Abuse and Mental Health Services Administration, "Recognizing and Treating Child Traumatic Stress," accessed September 25, 2020, https://www.samhsa.gov/child-trauma/recognizing-and-treating-child-traumatic-stress.

3. National Child Traumatic Stress Network, "How Early Childhood Trauma Is Unique."

CHAPTER 30. MEDICAL TRAUMA IN PARENTS

1. Julia Price et al., "Systematic Review: A Reevaluation and Update of the Integrative (Trajectory) Model of Pediatric Medical Traumatic Stress," *Journal of Pediatric Psychology* 41 (2016): 86–97, https://doi.org/10.1093/jpepsy/jsv074.

2. Anne E. Kazak et al., "Posttraumatic Stress Symptoms during Treatment in Parents of Children with Cancer," *Journal of Clinical Oncology* 23, no. 30 (2005): 7405–10, https://doi.org/10.1200/jco.2005.09.110.

3. Flaura Koplin Winston et al., "Acute Stress Disorder Symptoms in Children and Their Parents after Pediatric Traffic Injury," *Pediatrics* 109, no. 6 (2002): e90, https://doi.org/10.1542/peds.109.6.e90.

4. American Psychiatric Association, *Diagnostic and Statistical Manual of Mental Disorders: DSM-5* (Arlington, VA: American Psychiatric Association, 2013).

5. Laura E. Watkins, Kelsey R. Sprang, and Barbara O. Rothbaum, "Treating PTSD: A Review of Evidence-Based Psychotherapy Interventions," *Frontiers in Behavioral Neuroscience* 12 (2018): 258, https://dx.doi.org/10.3389/fnbeh.2018.00258.

Bibliography

Ageranioti-Bélanger, Stacey, Suzanne Brunet, Guy D'Anjou, Geneviève Tellier, Johanne Boivin, and Marie Gauthier. "Behaviour Disorders in Children with an Intellectual Disability." *Paediatrics and Child Health* 17, no. 2 (2012): 84–88. https://doi.org/10.1093/pch/17.2.84.

Alisic, Eva, Marian J. Jongmans, Floryt van Wesel, and Rolf J. Kleber. "Building Child Trauma Theory from Longitudinal Studies: A Meta-Analysis." *Clinical Psychology Review* 31, no. 5 (2011): 736–47. https://doi.org/10.1016/j.cpr.2011.03.001.

Allen, Karen M., Jim Blascovich, Joe Tomaka, and Robert M. Kelsey. "Presence of Human Friends and Pet Dogs as Moderators of Autonomic Responses to Stress in Women." *Journal of Personality and Social Psychology* 61 (1991): 582–89. https://psycnet.apa.org/doi/10.1037/0022-3514.61.4.582.

American Childhood Cancer Organization. "US Childhood Cancer Statistics." Accessed September 25, 2020. https://www.acco.org/us-childhood-cancer-statistics/.

American Medical Association. "Code of Medical Ethics Opinion 2.2.1." Accessed September 25, 2020. https://www.ama-assn.org/delivering-care/ethics/informed-consent.

American Psychiatric Association. *Diagnostic and Statistical Manual of Mental Disorders: DSM-5*. Arlington, VA: American Psychiatric Association, 2013.

Anderson, Lynda Lahti, Sheryl A. Larson, Sarah MapelLentz, and Jennifer Hall-Lande. "A Systematic Review of US Studies on the Prevalence of Intellectual or Developmental Disabilities Since 2000." *Intellectual and Devel-*

opment Disabilities 57, no. 5 (2019): 421–38. https://doi.org/10.1352/1934-9556-57.5.421.

Applied Behavior Analysis Programs Guide. "What Is Visual Scheduling." Accessed September 25, 2020. https://www.appliedbehavioranalysisprograms.com/faq/what-is-visual-scheduling/.

Autism Speaks Autism Treatment Network. "Visual Supports and Autism Spectrum Disorders." Accessed September 25, 2020. https://www.autismspeaks.org/sites/default/files/2018-08/Visual%20Supports%20Tool%20Kit.pdf.

Barnes, Andrew J., Marla E. Eisenberg, and Michael D. Resnick. "Suicide and Self-Injury among Children and Youth with Chronic Health Conditions." *Pediatrics* 125, no. 5 (2010): 889–95. https://doi.org/10.1542/peds.2009-1814.

Baumrind, Diana. "Effects of Authoritative Parental Control on Child Behavior." *Child Development* 37, no. 4 (1966): 887–907. https://psycnet.apa.org/doi/10.2307/1126611.

Béranger, Agathe, Charlotte Pierron, Laure de Saint Blanquat, and Hélène Chappuy. "Communication, informations et place des parents en réanimation polyvalente pédiatrique: Revue de la littérature [Communication, Information, and Roles of Parents in the Pediatric Intensive Care Unit: A Review Article]." *Archives de Pédiatrie* 24, no. 3 (2017): 265–72. https://doi.org/10.1016/j.arcped.2016.12.001.

Bethell, Christina D., Michael D. Kogan, Bonnie B. Strickland, Edward L. Schor, Julie Robertson, and Paul W. Newacheck. "A National and State Profile of Leading Health Problems and Health Care Quality for US Children: Key Insurance Disparities and Across-State Variations." *Academic Pediatrics* 11, suppl. 3 (2011): S22–33. https://doi.org/10.1016/j.acap.2010.08.011.

Biography.com. "What Was Albert Einstein's IQ?" Accessed September 25, 2020. https://www.biography.com/news/albert-einstein-iq.

Blackman, James A., Matthew J. Gurka, Kelly K. Gurka, and M. Norman Oliver. "Emotional, Developmental, and Behavioural Comorbidities of Children with Chronic Health Conditions." *Journal of Paediatrics and Child Health* 47, no. 10 (2011): 742–47. https://doi.org/10.1111/j.1440-1754.2011.02044.x.

Brenner, Maria, Margaret Pearl Treacy, Jonathan Drennan, and Gerard Fealty. "Nurses' Perceptions of the Practice of Restricting a Child for a Clinical Procedure." *Qualitative Health Research* 24, no. 8 (2014): 1080–89. https://dx.doi.org/10.1177/1049732314541332.

Brown, Brené. "The Wholehearted Parenting Manifesto." *HuffPost*. Updated November 28, 2012. https://www.huffpost.com/entry/wholehearted-parenting-manifesto_b_1923011.

"Caring." In *Oxford English Dictionary/Lexico*. Accessed September 23, 2020. https://www.lexico.com/en/definition/caring.

Centers for Disease Control and Prevention. "How to Use Rewards." Accessed September 25, 2020. https://www.cdc.gov/parents/essentials/consequences/rewards.html.

Centers for Disease Control and Prevention, National Center for Injury Prevention and Control. "Injury Prevention & Control: WISQARS™ Injury Data." Accessed September 25, 2020. https://www.cdc.gov/injury/wisqars/index.html.

Chambers, Christine T., Anne Taddio, Lindsay S. Uman, and C. Meghan McMurtry. "Psychological Interventions for Reducing Pain and Distress during Routine Childhood Immunizations: A Systematic Review." *Clinical Therapeutics* 31, suppl. 2 (2009): s77–s103. https://doi.org/10.1016/j.clinthera.2009.07.023.

Children's National Hospital. "Beyond the Spectrum: Visual Supports and Resources." Accessed September 25, 2020. https://childrensnational.org/departments/center-for-neuroscience-and-behavioral-medicine/programs-and-services/center-for-autism-spectrum-disorders/beyond-the-spectrum/visual-supports-and-resources.

Cobos, Briana, Kelly Haskard-Zolnierek, and Krista Howard. "White Coat Hypertension: Improving the Patient-Health Care Practitioner Relationship." *Psychology Research and Behavior Management* 8 (2015): 133–41. https://doi.org/10.2147/prbm.s61192.

Cohen, Lindsey L., Ronald L. Blount, and Georgia Panopoulos. "Nurse Coaching and Cartoon Distraction: An Effective and Practical Intervention to Reduce Child, Parent, and Nurse Distress during Immunizations." *Journal of Pediatric Psychology* 22, no. 3 (1997): 355–70. https://doi.org/10.1093/jpepsy/22.3.355.

Coley, Rebekah Levine, Alicia Doyle Lynch, and Melissa Kull. "Early Exposure to Environmental Chaos and Children's Physical and Mental Health." *Early Childhood Research Quarterly* 32, no. 3 (2015): 94–104. https://dx.doi.org/10.1016/j.ecresq.2015.03.001.

Committee to Evaluate the Supplemental Security Income Disability Program for Children with Mental Disorders. "Clinical Characteristics of Intellectual Disabilities." In *Mental Disorders and Disabilities among Low-Income Children*, edited by Thomas F. Boat and Joel T. Wu. Washington, DC: National Academies Press, 2015. https://www.ncbi.nlm.nih.gov/books/NBK332877/.

Devanarayana, Niranga Manjuri, Sachith Mettananda, Chathurangi Liyanarachchi, Navoda Nanayakkara, Niranjala Mendis, Nimnadi Perera, and Shaman Rajindrajith. "Abdominal Pain–Predominant Functional Gastrointestinal Diseases in Children and Adolescents: Prevalence, Symptomatology, and Association with Emotional Stress." *Journal of Pediatric Gastroenterology and Nutrition* 53, no. 6 (2011): 659–65. https://doi.org/10.1097/mpg.0b013e3182296033.

"Deviation IQ." In *A Dictionary of Psychology*. Accessed September 23, 2020. https://www.oxfordreference.com/view/10.1093/oi/authority.20110803095714395.

Finkelhor, David, Richard Ormrod, and Heather A. Turner. "Lifetime Assessment of Poly-Victimization in a National Sample of Children and Youth." *Child Abuse and Neglect* 33, no. 7 (2009): 403–11. https://doi.org/10.1016/j.chiabu.2008.09.012.

Ginsburg, Kenneth R., and the Committee on Communications and the Committee on Psychosocial Aspects of Child and Family Health of the American Academy of Pediatrics. "The Importance of Play in Promoting Healthy Child Development and Maintaining Strong Parent-Child Bonds." *Pediatrics* 119, no. 1 (2007): 182–91. https://doi.org/10.1542/peds.2006-2697.

Graboyes, Robert. "Medical Paternalism in Many Guises." Mercatus Center at George Mason University. July 6, 2017. https://www.mercatus.org/essays/medical-paternalism-many-guises.

Graboyes, Robert F., and Eric Topol. *Anatomy and Atrophy of Medical Paternalism*. Arlington, VA: Mercatus Research, Mercatus Center at George Mason University, 2017. Accessed September 25, 2020. https://www.mercatus.org/system/files/mercatus-graboyes-medical-paternalism-v3_1.pdf.

Hsieh, Pei-Hsuan. "Positive Reinforcement." In *Encyclopedia of Child Behavior and Development*, edited by Sam Goldstein and Jack A. Naglieri. Boston: Springer, 2011. https://doi.org/10.1007/978-0-387-79061-9_2916.

Jones, Alyssa C., Nancy Kassam-Adams, Jeffrey A. Ciesla, Lamia P. Barakat, and Meghan L. Marsac. "A Prospective Examination of Child Avoidance Coping and Parental Coping Assistance after Pediatric Injury: A Mixed-Methods Approach." *Journal of Pediatric Psychology* 44, no. 8 (2019): 914–23. https://doi.org/10.1093/jpepsy/jsz016.

Kakkar, Mayank, Astha Wahi, Radhika Thakkar, Iqra Vohra, and Arvind Kumar Shukla. "Prevalence of Dental Anxiety in 10–14 Years Old Children and Its Implications." *Journal of Dental Anesthesia and Pain Medicine* 16, no. 3 (2016): 199–202. https://doi.org/10.17245/jdapm.2016.16.3.199.

Kazak, Anne E., C. Alexandra Boeving, Melissa A. Alderfer, Wei-Ting Hwang, and Anne Reilly. "Posttraumatic Stress Symptoms during Treatment in Parents of Children with Cancer." *Journal of Clinical Oncology* 23, no. 30 (2005): 7405–10. https://doi.org/10.1200/jco.2005.09.110.

Kazak, Anne E., Nancy Kassam-Adams, Stephanie Schneider, Nataliya Zelikovsky, Melissa A. Alderfer, and Mary Rourke. "An Integrative Model of Pediatric Medical Traumatic Stress." *Journal of Pediatric Psychology* 31, no. 4 (2006): 343–55. https://doi.org/10.1093/jpepsy/jsj054.

Kepreotes, Elizabeth, Diana Keatinge, and Teresa Elizabeth Stone. "The Experience of Parenting Children with Chronic Health Conditions: A New Reality." *Journal of Nursing and Healthcare of Chronic Illness* 2, no. 1 (2010): 51–62. http://dx.doi.org/10.1111/j.1752-9824.2010.01047.x.

Kertes, Darlene A., Jingwen Liu, Nathan J. Hall, Natalie A. Hadad, Clive D. L. Wynne, and Samarth S. Bhatt. "Effect of Pet Dogs on Children's Perceived Stress and Cortisol Stress Response." *Social Development* 26, no. 2 (2017): 382–401. https://doi.org/10.1111/sode.12203.

Koller, Donna, and Ran D. Goldman. "Distraction Techniques for Children Undergoing Procedures: A Critical Review of Pediatric Research." *Journal of Pediatric Nursing* 27, no. 6 (2012): 652–81. https://doi.org/10.1016/j.pedn.2011.08.001.

Landry, Susan H., Karen E. Smith, Paul R. Swank, Mike A. Assel, and Sonya Vellet. "Does Early Responsive Parenting Have a Special Importance for Children's Development or Is Consistency across Early Childhood Necessary?" *Developmental Psychology* 37, no. 3 (2001): 387–403. https://doi.org/10.1037/0012-1649.37.3.387.

Lanius, Ulrich F., Sandra L. Paulsen, and Frank M. Corrigan, eds. "Threat and Safety: The Neurobiology of Active and Passive Defense Responses." In *Neurobiology and the Treatment of Traumatic Dissociation: Toward an Embodied Self*, 29–50. New York: Springer, 2014.

Maccoby, Eleanor E., and John A. Martin. "Socialization in the Context of the Family: Parent-Child Interaction." In *Handbook of Child Psychology: Socialization, Personality and Social Development*, 1–101, 4th ed., edited by E. M. Hetherington (vol. ed.) and Paul H. Mussen (series ed.). New York: Wiley, 1983.

Marsac, Meghan L., Christine Kindler, Danielle Weiss, and Lindsay Ragsdale. "Let's Talk about It: Supporting Family Communication during End-of-Life Care of Pediatric Patients." *Journal of Palliative Medicine* 21, no. 6 (2018): 862–78. https://doi.org/10.1089/jpm.2017.0307.

Marsac, Meghan L., and Jeanne B. Funk. "Relationships among Psychological Functioning, Dental Anxiety, Pain Perception, and Coping in Children and Adolescents." *Journal of Dentistry for Children* 75, no. 3 (2008): 243–51.

Marsac, Meghan L., Jeffrey Ciesla, Lamia P. Barakat, Aimee K. Hildenbrand, Douglas L. Delahanty, Keith Widaman, Flaura K. Winston, et al. "The Role of Appraisals and Coping in Predicting Posttraumatic Stress Following Pediatric Injury." *Psychological Trauma: Theory, Research, Practice, and Policy* 8, no. 4 (2016): 495–503. https://dx.doi.org/10.1037/tra0000116.

Marsac, Meghan L., Nancy Kassam-Adams, Douglas L. Delahanty, Jeffrey Ciesla, Danielle Weiss, Keith F. Widaman, and Lamia P. Barakat. "An Initial Application of a Bio-Psycho-Social Framework to Predict Posttraumatic Stress Following Pediatric Injury." *Health Psychology* 36, no. 8 (2017): 787–96. https://dx.doi.org/10.1037%2Fhea0000508.

Marsac, Meghan L., Nancy Kassam-Adams, Douglas L. Delahanty, Keith Widaman, and Lamia P. Barakat. "Posttraumatic Stress Following Acute Medical Trauma in Children: A Proposed Model of Bio-Psycho-Social Processes during the Peri-Trauma Period." *Clinical Child and Family Psychology Review* 17, no. 4 (2014): 1–13. https://dx.doi.org/10.1007/s10567-014-0174-2.

May, Kathleen M. "Searching for Normalcy: Mothers' Caregiving for Low Birthweight Infants." *Pediatric Nursing* 23, no. 1 (1997): 17–20.

McKenzie, Katherine, Meagan Milton, Glenys Smith, and Hélène Ouellette-Kuntz. "Systematic Review of the Prevalence and Incidence of Intellectual Disabilities: Current Trends and Issues." *Current Developmental Disorders Report* 3 (June 2016): 104–15. https://doi.org/10.1007/s40474-016-0085-7.

Meadows, Amy L., and Meghan L. Marsac. "Early Life Trauma and Diabetes Management: An Under-Recognized Phenomenon in Transition-Age Youth." *Clinical Diabetes* 38, no. 1 (2020): 93–95. https://doi.org/10.2337/cd19-0012.

National Child Traumatic Stress Network. "How Early Childhood Trauma Is Unique." Accessed September 25, 2020. https://www.nctsn.org/what-is-child-trauma/trauma-types/early-childhood-trauma/effects.

National Institute of Mental Health Information Resource Center. "5 Things You Should Know about Stress." Accessed September 25, 2020. https://www.nimh.nih.gov/health/publications/stress/index.shtml.

National Institutes of Health, National Center for Complementary and Integrative Health. "Relaxation Techniques for Health." Accessed September 25, 2020. https://www.nccih.nih.gov/health/relaxation-techniques-for-health.

National Organization for Rare Disorders. Home page. Accessed September 25, 2020. https://rarediseases.org/get-involved/donate-now/give/35-years-growing/.

Park, Myonghwa, Thi-Thanh-Tinh Giap, Mihyun Lee, Hyun Jeong, Miri Jeong, and Younghye Go. "Patient- and Family-Centered Care Interventions for Improving the Quality of Health Care: A Review of Systematic Reviews." *International Journal of Nursing Studies* 87 (2018): 69–83. https://doi.org/10.1016/j.ijnurstu.2018.07.006.

Pew Research Center. "Parenting in America: Outlook, Worries, Aspirations Are Strongly Linked to Financial Situation." December 17, 2015. https://www.pewsocialtrends.org/wp-content/uploads/sites/3/2015/12/2015-12-17_parenting-in-america_FINAL.pdf.

Price, Julia, Nancy Kassam-Adams, Melissa A. Alderfer, Jennifer Christofferson, and Anne E. Kazak. "Systematic Review: A Reevaluation and Update of the Integrative (Trajectory) Model of Pediatric Medical Traumatic Stress." *Journal of Pediatric Psychology* 41 (2016): 86–97. https://doi.org/10.1093/jpepsy/jsv074.

Raina, Parminder, Maureen O'Donnell, Peter Rosenbaum, Jamie Brehaut, Stephen D. Walter, Dianne Russell, Marilyn Swinton, et al. "The Health and Well-Being of Caregivers of Children with Cerebral Palsy." *Pediatrics* 115, no. 6 (2015): 626–36. https://doi.org/10.1542/peds.2004-1689.

Rancourt, Kate M., Jill M. Chorney, and Zeev Kain. "Children's Immediate Postoperative Distress and Mothers' and Fathers' Touch Behaviors."

Journal of Pediatric Psychology 40, no. 10 (2015): 1115–23. https://dx.doi.org/10.1093/jpepsy/jsv069.

Schechter, Neil L., William T. Zempsky, Lindsey L. Cohen, Patrick J. McGrath, C. Meghan McMurtry, and Nancy S. Bright. "Pain Reduction during Pediatric Immunizations: Evidence-Based Review and Recommendations." *Pediatrics* 119 (2007): e1184–98. https://doi.org/10.1542/peds.2006-1107.

Seresinhe, Chanuki Illushka, Tobias Preis, George MacKerron, and Helen Susannah Moat. "Happiness Is Greater in More Scenic Locations." *Scientific Reports* 9 (2019): 4498. https://doi.org/10.1038/s41598-019-40854-6.

Substance Abuse and Mental Health Services Administration. "Recognizing and Treating Child Traumatic Stress." Accessed September 25, 2020. https://www.samhsa.gov/child-trauma/recognizing-and-treating-child-traumatic-stress.

Taddio, Anna, Moshe Ipp, Suganthan Thivakaran, Ali Jamal, Chaitya Parikh, Sarah Smart, Julia Sovran, et al. "Survey of the Prevalence of Immunization Non-Compliance Due to Needle Fears in Children and Adults." *Vaccine* 30, no. 32 (2012): 4807–12. https://doi.org/10.1016/j.vaccine.2012.05.011.

Tsao, Jennie C. I., Qian Lu, Su C. Kim, and Lonnie K. Zeltzer. "Relationships among Anxious Symptomatology, Anxiety Sensitivity and Laboratory Pain Responsivity in Children." *Cognitive Behaviour Therapy* 35, no. 4 (2006): 207–15. https://doi.org/10.1080/16506070600898272.

Ulrich, Roger, Xiaobo Quan, Craig Zimring, Anjali Joseph, and Ruchi Choudhary. *The Role of the Physical Environment in the 21st Century Hospital, Report to The Center for Health Design for the Designing the 21st Century Hospital Project*. Princeton, NJ: Robert Wood Johnson Foundation, 2004. https://www.healthdesign.org/system/files/Ulrich_Role%20of%20Physical_2004.pdf.

U.S. Department of Education, National Center for Education Statistics. "Table 204.30: Children 3 to 21 Years Old Served under Individuals with Disabilities Education Act (IDEA), Part B, by Type of Disability; Selected Years 1976–77 through 2017–18." *Digest of Education Statistics, 2018*. Washington, DC: National Center for Education Statistics, 2020. https://nces.ed.gov/programs/digest/d18/tables/dt18_204.30.asp.

Vardar-Yagli, Naciye, Melda Saglam, Deniz Inal-Ince, Ebru Calik-Kutukcu, Hulya Arikan, Sema Savci, Ugur Ozcelik, et al. "Hospitalization of Children with Cystic Fibrosis Adversely Affects Mothers' Physical Activity, Sleep Quality, and Psychological Status." *Journal of Child and Family Studies* 26, no. 3 (2017): 800–9. https://doi.org/10.1007/s10826-016-0593-4.

Watkins, Laura E., Kelsey R. Sprang, and Barbara O. Rothbaum. "Treating PTSD: A Review of Evidence-Based Psychotherapy Interventions." *Frontiers in Behavioral Neuroscience* 12 (2018): 258. https://dx.doi.org/10.3389/fnbeh.2018.00258.

Winston, Flaura Koplin, Nancy Kassam-Adams, Cara Vivarelli-O'Neill, Julian Ford, Elana Newman, Chiara Baxt, Perry Stafford, et al. "Acute Stress Disorder Symptoms in Children and Their Parents after Pediatric Traffic Injury." *Pediatrics* 109, no. 6 (2002): e90. https://doi.org/10.1542/peds.109.6.e90.

Zahran, Hatice S., Cathy M. Bailey, Scott A. Damon, Paul L. Garbe, and Patrick N. Breysse. "Vital Signs: Asthma in Children—United States, 2001–2016." *Morbidity and Mortality Weekly Report* 67 (2018): 149–55. http://dx.doi.org/10.15585/mmwr.mm6705e1.

Index

Page references for figures are italicized.

About the Authors

Meghan L. Marsac, PhD, is a pediatric psychologist and a tenured associate professor at the University of Kentucky and Kentucky Children's Hospital. Dr. Marsac is a leader in the field of pediatric medical trauma, having published more than fifty-five academic articles and nine chapters on this topic. Her primary professional goal is to improve the experience of living with medical conditions for children and families. Her work is represented in leading medical journals such as *JAMA Pediatrics* and *Pediatrics* and leading health psychology journals such as the *Journal of Pediatric Psychology* and *Health Psychology*. Dr. Marsac currently serves on the editorial board of the *Journal of Pediatric Psychology* and *Journal of Traumatic Stress*. Dr. Marsac has also given hundreds of talks on understanding and promoting adjustment to injury and illness in children and their families. She is CEO of the Cellie Coping Company (www.celliecopingcompany.com), which has distributed over two thousand coping kits to families of children with medical conditions. In addition, Dr. Marsac specializes in training medical teams in the implementation of trauma-informed medical care. Clinically, Dr. Marsac implements evidence-based practices to facilitate families' management of medical treatment and emotional adjustment to challenging diagnoses and medical procedures.

Melissa J. Hogan, JD, is a consultant on clinical trial design and patient outcome measures in rare and neurodegenerative disorders. She also serves as a patient representative to the U.S. Food and Drug Administration and on the FDA/CTTI Patient Engagement Collaborative with the goal of incorporating the patient voice into the processes for U.S. drug and device evaluation and approval. She was previously the cofounder and president of Project Alive, a leading research and advocacy foundation for patients with Hunter syndrome, and prior to that she worked as a corporate health care attorney. She is published in journals such as *Molecular Genetics and Metabolism* and is a requested speaker at industry conferences on topics ranging from patient advocacy to clinical trial design. Her interest and research on medical trauma was sparked by her participation with her youngest son in a clinical trial for over ten years, along with weekly infusions and ten specialists.

CPSIA information can be obtained
at www.ICGtesting.com
Printed in the USA
LVHW092234240821
695914LV00014B/23